75p

THE *SHE*
BOOK OF
FAMILY HEALTH

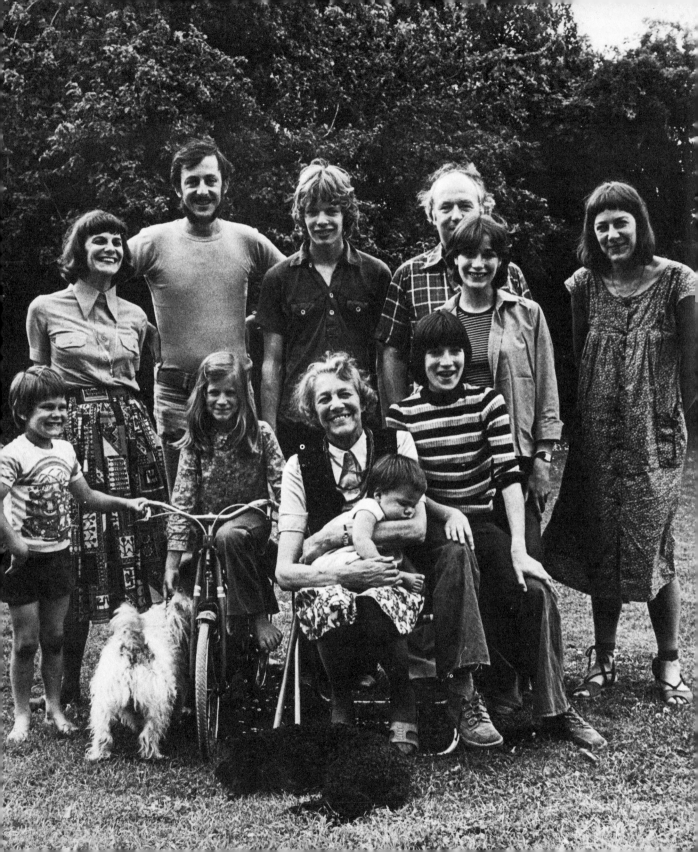

THE *SHE*
BOOK OF
FAMILY HEALTH

THE MEDICAL ADVICE
AND INFORMATION
YOUR FAMILY NEEDS

Dr David Delvin

BOOK CLUB ASSOCIATES
LONDON

This edition published 1983 by
Book Club Associates
by arrangement with Arthur Barker Ltd
91 Clapham High Street, London SW4 7TA
and Ebury Press
National Magazine House, 72 Broadwick Street, London W1V 2BP

Set in Great Britain by
Advanced Filmsetters (Glasgow) Ltd
Printed and bound in Great Britain by
The University Press, Cambridge

CONTENTS

Introduction   7

The NHS, Your Doctor and You   9

A Guide to a Healthy Life
General good health   13
Good eating   14
Good sleep and relaxation   15
Good love—and good sex   15
Good sense about smoking and drinking   16

The Seven Ages of Man (and Woman)
I The first twelve months   18
II The playschool age   20
III The younger school child   22
IV Puberty and the teenage years   23
V The younger adult   25
VI The middle years   26
VII Growing older   27

A Three Part A–Z
A–Z of Parts of the Body   30
A–Z of Conditions and Diseases   42
A–Z of Emergencies   133

Index   142

Acknowledgements   144

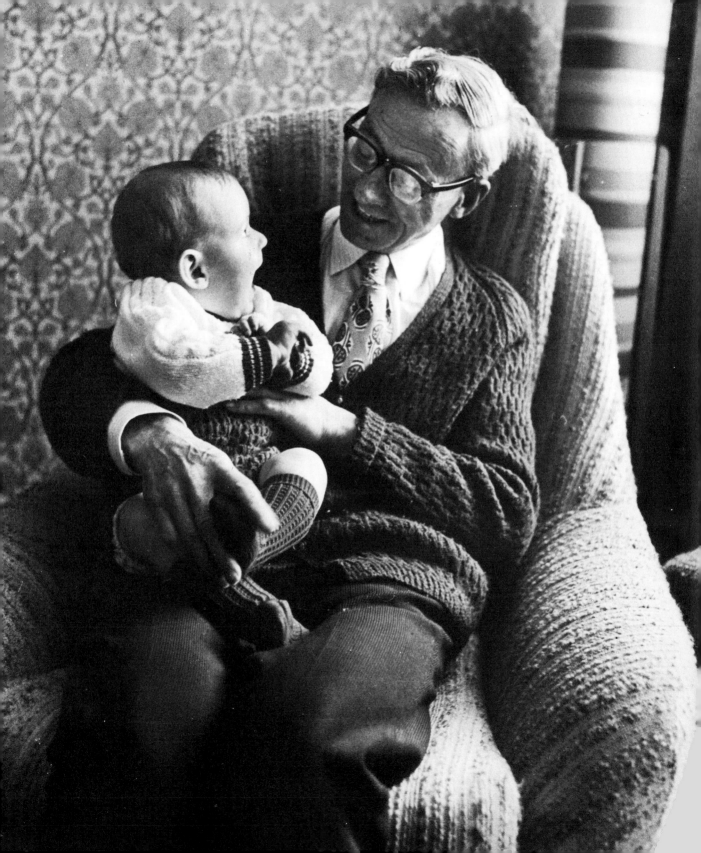

INTRODUCTION

Everybody wants the best possible health for themselves—and for their families.

Yet, unfortunately, most people *don't* know a great deal about their bodies.

Here's a simple illustration of that fact. Several years ago, I twice organized and judged a 'Health Contest' for BBC-TV's popular *Generation Game*.

The idea of this particular competition was quite simple. On four podia stood two all-in wrestlers and two beauty queens. Male contestants had to stick 'health labels' (with the names of organs or diseases) on the beauty queens—while of course female contestants had to stick similar labels on the all-in wrestlers.

The results were absolutely ludicrous! People thought that their livers were up near their left shoulders; they thought their kidneys were where their lungs are, and *vice versa*.

I need hardly tell you where they thought you get pyelitis (which is actually a kidney condition, as you'll see from this book).

And when it came to the bone called the coccyx—well, I have an abiding memory of a middle-aged lady slapping the relevant sticker right in the centre front of an all-in wrestler's trunks. (To his credit, he never blinked an eyelid—a remarkable tribute to the stoicism of the wrestling profession.)

All very jokey, I know. But there's a serious message.

People's lack of knowledge about their bodies and their health is bad for them.

To take just a few examples which are of great concern to the Health Education Council:

● At least half the kids in the country haven't been fully immunized—so some of them still die of polio, diphtheria, whooping cough or even measles.

● 30,000 people a year are dying quite needlessly of our commonest cancer (yes, *lung* cancer) because the public still doesn't really understand that smoking causes it.

● A far larger number of people are dying of heart attacks, believed now to be caused mainly by unhealthy habits—again, including smoking—and a poor choice of diet.

● 140,000 women a year are having abortions—many of them because they and their partners don't know enough about their own bodies to use the very, very effective methods of contraception which we now have available.

● Each winter, hundreds of older people die because they and their relatives don't know how to avoid hypothermia.

Sorry to sound so gloomy! There *are* more cheerful examples of public lack of knowledge about the human body. For instance, there's the woman who says: 'I'm going in for that operation: *you* know—they call it the hysterical rectum'.

Anyway, I hope that *The SHE Book of Family Health* will help you and your family to the best possible understanding of your bodies—and to good health!

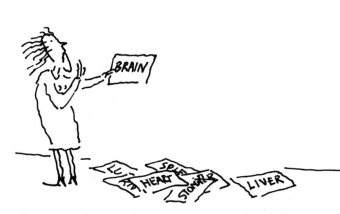

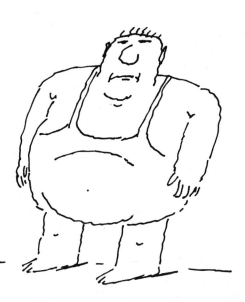

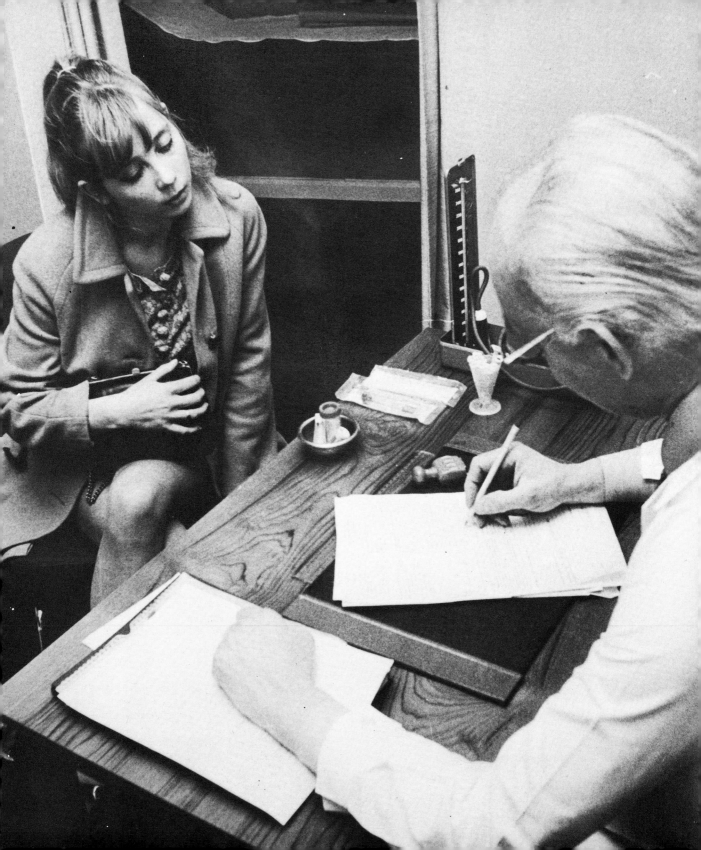

THE NHS, YOUR DOCTOR AND YOU

No, this isn't going to be a full guide to the vast complexities of NHS bureaucracy!

In fact, the National Health Service has just been re-organized (yet again) in an attempt to make it more efficient. What will come out of that re-organization, heaven alone knows. But certain basic things about the way the NHS is organized will remain the same—and it will pay you to know about them.

The NHS is a vast 'enterprise', employing well over a million people, and run by the Department of Health and Social Security in London, and the Scottish Home and Health Department in Edinburgh.

It's paid for mainly from taxation—not from National Insurance stamps, as people often imagine. With certain restrictions, it's FREE to everyone who lives in Britain.

It may not be 'the envy of the world', as politicians so often and so boringly claim—but it does on the whole provide a very good service for the person who is taken suddenly ill. If you have a coronary or go into premature labour or get run over by a motorbike, then the NHS will look after you—and look after you FREE.

In great contrast to the situation in so many other countries, neither the ambulance drivers nor the nurses nor anyone else is going to be remotely interested in the state of your bank balance, or whether you carry health insurance.

Unfortunately, the NHS *isn't* so good on long-term things. The services for chronic physical and mental disability and for the elderly are not exactly fantastic, and the enormous waiting lists to get into hospital (currently standing at around 700,000 people) bear witness to the fact that the Health Service is really far from perfect.

Of course, the fact is that it can *never* be perfect—because to pour money into it to make it better is like tipping gold into a bottomless pit.

However, there are two things *you* can do:

● When you spot serious deficiencies in the NHS, you can *complain*: this section will tell you how.

● You can also make sure that you understand the basic workings of the NHS—so that you and your family can use it to the best advantage.

BASIC WORKINGS OF THE NHS

There are really three great divisions of the National Health Service:

● The Family Doctor and Dentist Service
● The Hospital Service
● The Community Health Services

Let's see how they all work—and also what you should do if you have a genuine complaint against the way these services have treated you or your family.

The Family Doctor and Dentist Service

We'll leave the dental service on one side for a moment and concentrate on the *family doctor* or general practitioner.

This is the man (or woman) with whom you're most likely to have contact in your dealings with the Health Service. That's especially true if you've got young children—for babies, toddlers and younger schoolchildren are more likely to need a GP's advice at some time. So too are the elderly, of course.

So it's worth selecting your GP *carefully*. Some are *very* good, most are *pretty* good, and a few—it's generally admitted—are just plain *awful*. Therefore, make sure you get a good one!

How? Well, when you move to a new area it's best to ask around; enquire from your neighbours or local shopkeepers about which family doctors in the area have the best reputation. Bear in mind that the person who may know most about the local GPs is probably the local chemist.

If you go to your post office, you can ask to have a look at a *list* of general practitioners. But, unfortunately, this just gives you names, addresses, and surgery times. However, it should also indicate (by means of a large 'C') whether a doctor is willing to prescribe contraception or not—a matter of some importance to young (and middle-aged!) adults. In fact, the vast majority of GPs do at least prescribe the Pill.

When you've selected some possible names of GPs, I'd suggest that the next thing is to ring up their surgeries *and see if they've got any room on their lists*. Unfortunately, many family doctors simply don't have any room for more patients.

Next, it may well be worth your while to go and look at the practice premises, and see what it's like. You may prefer the small one-man surgery—or you may like the idea of a large modern-looking health centre, with several doctors and plenty of health visitors, social workers and so on bustling around the place.

A few brave souls actually ask for an *interview* with a prospective GP, and there's no reason why you shouldn't do this. Some doctors will refuse to be interviewed—but a surprisingly large number won't, since it can be very useful for both 'sides' to get to know each other.

Once you've decided on your GP and 'signed on' with him, then you're his patient, and he's responsible for the care of you and your family, until such time as you move to another district. (If you ever decide to *change* your GP, look in your medical card where you'll find the procedure described.)

Can I here say one word on behalf of the family doctors? It's not generally realized that they *do* have an enormous workload. On average, they see about 43 patients every day—with many of those patients posing all sorts of difficult physical and psychological problems.

That's why the busy GP sees one patient *every six minutes*, which certainly isn't very much time—especially when you've allowed for a few 'good mornings' and a bit of dressing and undressing!

So when you go and see your family doctor, you certainly shouldn't hang about discussing the weather (which some people do!). But if there's something really worrying you, a good GP will ALWAYS find time to deal with it—even if it means bringing you back at some later time to discuss it in full.

A few further points which will help your relationship with your GP:

● If you need a home visit, try to ring his surgery before 10 am to ask him for one.

● Don't expect a prescription from him every time you see him—often a chat and some advice is a helluva lot better than drugs.

● *Don't* try and manipulate him into prescribing drugs which YOU think are best for you—let's face it, he knows 100 times more about medicines than you do.

● If you've got an appointment for one person, *don't* try and get other members of the family seen 'in the same slot': remember, the unfortunate GP is basically trying to keep to that awful 'six minutes a patient' schedule.

Complaints: if you feel you have a complaint about your GP, it may be a good idea to write to him first; a lot of troubles between patients and GPs are really due to silly misunderstandings caused by tiredness or lack of communication, and are best sorted out between you and your doctor if at all possible.

But if things are more serious than that, then you can complain to your *Family Practitioner Committee* (address in your medical card) who run the local general practitioner services.

It's also possible to raise complaints with your local *Community Health Council* (address in the phone book). The CHC is supposed to be the 'consumers' watchdog' in the NHS, and though it has no executive powers, an effective CHC can do a good deal to sort out problems.

In really serious matters, you can complain to the *Health Service Ombudsman* (your local Citizens' Advice Bureau will tell you how to do this). But he will not rule on matters of doctors' clinical judgement of an illness.

If you feel that you have a *legal* grievance against a doctor (in other words that you could sue him or her for damages) then your only course is to consult a solicitor. If you aren't well off, this can be done through the *Legal Aid Scheme*.

In my view, only if you feel that a doctor's behaviour amounts to serious professional misconduct (for instance, sleeping with a patient or gross neglect of duty) should you complain to the *General Medical Council* (GMC). There is no point in complaining to the BMA, which is a different organization from the GMC and has no disciplinary function.

But I come back to the fact that—as the Deputy Health Ombudsman recently told me—*most disputes between doctor and patient are really due to misunderstandings and failure of communication.*

So it's really much better, if at all possible, to try and sort out disagreements *personally* with your doctor, and if you *can't* do so, change your doctor.

The Family Dentist. Under the NHS, people *aren't* 'signed up' with one family dentist in the same way as they are with a family doctor.

However, there's much to be said for having *one* dentist who looks after your children's teeth (and yours!) for some years at a time—especially if you can find a dentist who's keen on PREVENTION of dental disease, rather than just treating it when it occurs.

But you and your family can go to any dentist you want to—provided he'll see you. Bear in mind that an awful lot of dentists have cut down on their NHS work, *so make very sure that the dentist has accepted you on the Health Service rather than privately.* You don't want a bill for £200 when you think you've been treated on the NHS!

The Hospital Service

You and your family can come into contact with the Hospital Service in two different ways. These are:

● When you're 'referred' by your GP to see an NHS consultant (*i.e.* a specialist).

● When you go 'off your own bat' to a Casualty (Accident & Emergency) Department.

BEING REFERRED BY YOUR GP. In general, you simply can't go and get a specialist's opinion without a referral letter from your GP. This may seen a bit restrictive, but there are good reasons for it—one being that in countries where the 'GP referral' system doesn't operate, all kinds of muddles occur, with patients being treated with one lot of drugs by a GP, and with another lot by a specialist.

There are a few exceptions to the rule: for instance, you can go to a Family Planning Clinic or to a VD Clinic *without* a GP's letter (and, as mentioned below, you can often go to Casualty without one).

But normally, hospitals just will not see you or your family without a family doctor's letter. Happily, a good GP is only too willing to write such a note when it is genuinely necessary.

GOING TO A CASUALTY (ACCIDENT & EMERGENCY) DEPARTMENT. In cases of genuine emergency, such as bad cuts, head injuries, broken bones and other trauma, you have the option of going to your local Accident & Emergency Department.

They will also see cases of sudden illness—for instance, if someone collapses with chest or abdominal pain, or if someone is found unconscious.

But they do tend to turn away patients who they feel should be treated by their own GPs—say, people with skin rashes and so on. If you're in doubt as to whether to go to your GP or to an 'A & E' Department, you could ring up first and ask.

Unfortunately, the number of Accident & Emergency Departments in Britain has been cut down a lot recently (on the dubious 'big is beautiful' theory of centralization).

So don't fall into the common trap of setting off for a hospital assuming that it's got a Casualty Department: most don't these days. Again, if in doubt, ring first.

COMPLAINTS. If you want to make a complaint about a hospital, begin by writing to the hospital administrator. If you have no joy, contact your local CHC (see above) or the NHS Ombudsman.

The Community Health Service
The Community Health Services are really too vast and amorphous to describe in full here, but basically they're the services which are run by your local authority.

From the family point of view, the most important Community Services are those provided by the Child Health Clinics, by Health Visitors, by District Nurses, by Social Workers, by Community Midwives, and by the School Medical Service. I'll be referring to most of these in the course of the book.

But in a nutshell, if your child is born at home he or she will probably be delivered by a Community Midwife. Even if you're delivered in hospital and *then* go home, the Community Midwife will be responsible for looking after him for the first 14 days. After that, the Health Visitor will help you with any problems.

During his babyhood and toddler years, you can take him to a Child Health Clinic (Infant Welfare Clinic) at regular intervals for such things as weighing, immunization and advice on feeding. And when he gets to school, the School Medical Service will oversee such matters as his immunizations—and whether he gets nits in his hair!

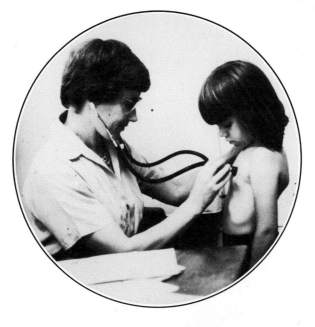

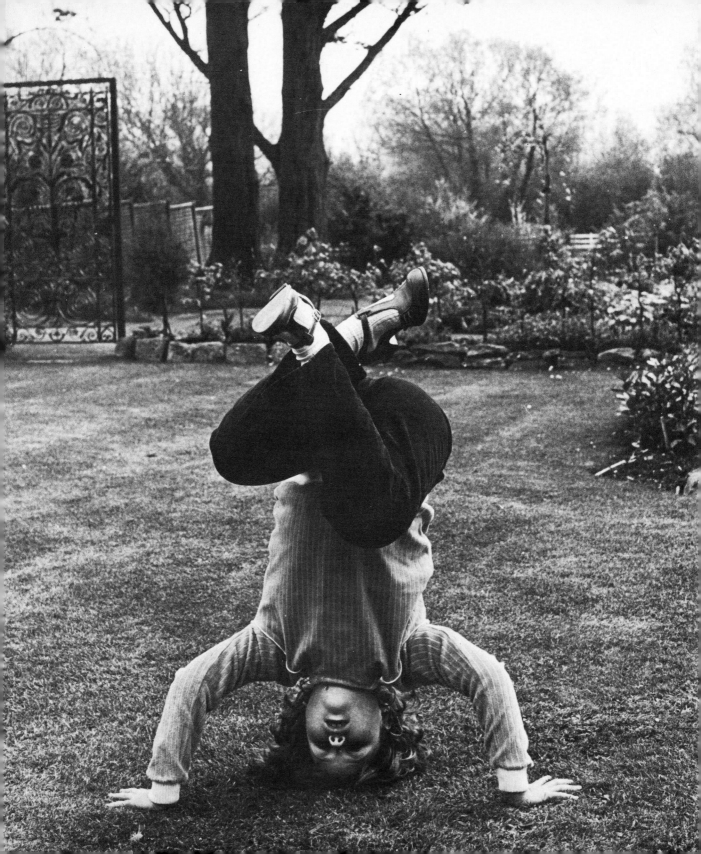

A GUIDE TO A HEALTHY LIFE

GENERAL GOOD HEALTH

What actually is complete good health? I suppose you could say that it's a state that no human being could possibly expect to achieve during his or her entire lifetime—at least for more than a few weeks or months at a time.

Why not? Because we are surrounded by threats to our health. Germs and pollutants are literally almost everywhere, and it's inevitable that some of them are going to affect us in some way at some time.

Also, we're all born with slight defects in our make-up. It may be only an allergy or an easily upset tummy, or it may be something more significant, like a tendency to arthritis or to high blood pressure. So, as no man or woman is completely perfect, it's not surprising that sometimes our workings do run into a bit of trouble.

That's why minor illnesses of one sort or another do occur pretty frequently. It's rather surprising that studies show that the average person has some episode of passing ill-health every two or three weeks!

If that seems staggering, then ask around at your office or workplace. You'll find that around half the people there will remember some kind of illness during the last fortnight. Perhaps a cough, or hay fever, or a sore throat, or a bad headache, or period pain, or piles, or a stiff shoulder, or tennis elbow.

If you become fit and healthy, the number of such minor problems will get less, but they won't go away altogether. Even a person who is 'A1' in health by anybody's standards, is going to suffer these minor pinpricks in life from time to time.

So being in 'good health' doesn't mean that you *never* have any minor illnesses at all. What it really means is that your body and mind are in the fittest possible condition to cope with the stresses and strains of life.

Are you in that sort of shape? If so, then you're in a tiny, tiny minority.

If you're not sure whether you're in that sort of shape, then do this little test I've worked out. Write in your scores, tot them up at the end, and then see how you rate:—

SCORE

Pinch the flesh on your tummy (just by the navel) between the finger and thumb. If you can't really pick up any fat, you score 4 points. One little roll of fat? 2 points. More than that? No points at all. _____

Do you get at least some exercise each day? 4 points for a lot of exercise, 2 points for moderate exercise, no points for 'none'. _____

Do you play some sort of active sport as well? 4 points for 'yes'; no points for 'no'. _____

Do you get backache or neckache? 2 points for 'never', 1 point for 'sometimes', no points for 'yes'. _____

How many average flights of stairs could you walk up without getting breathless? Count 2 points for each flight. _____

Do you smoke? Count 6 points for 'no'; 1 point if you smoke five per day or less; and minus 2 if you smoke more than five. _____

Do you drink more than about four pints of beer, or about four double whiskies or gin or around a bottle of wine a day? 4 points for 'no'; no points for 'yes'. _____

How many pills of any sort (excepting the contraceptive pill) have you taken in the last twenty four hours? Score minus 2 for each. _____

TOTAL _____

How did you get on? I must admit that the quiz is just a very, very rough test of fitness and health. But if you scored 20 or more, then you're very likely to be in pretty good nick!

If you totted up between 15 and 19, then you're probably not in bad shape, but there's some room for improvement. 10 to 14? Not too good. Five to nine? Oh dear! Under five? If you're not already seeing your doctor, then perhaps you should do so. If you got a minus total for any reason (unless your score has been pulled down by taking a lot of aspirin for a bad cold) then you should certainly be having medical advice.

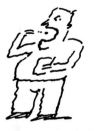

GOOD EATING

You've heard the slogan: 'You are what you eat'. And it's perfectly true. We start out in life consisting of about seven pounds of various bits of material which come from what our mother ate during her pregnancy—and, from then on, every last molecule of our bodies is formed due to what we take in through our mouths.

If we eat a lot of 'junk foods' (which is precisely what a lot of people, especially youngsters, do eat) then it's quite inevitable that our bodies will be in pretty rotten shape. Indeed, in some ways it's surprising that the human body manages to cope as well as it does with the sheer *rubbish* that Western man and woman shovel into it!

So how do we make sure that we get a decent, all round diet that will help to keep us healthy? Like most doctors, I'm not a health-food fiend, nor a vegetarian, though I do think that health-food people (and vegetarians) have some very good ideas, even if they are sometimes mixed up with some slightly daft ones.

But let's make clear from the start that, in the view of nearly all doctors, it *isn't* necessary for normal fit non-pregnant people to take vitamin pills or any other odd dietary additives in order to be healthy. The only exception to this rule occurs if you happen to be suffering from a genuine deficiency disease. And though people spend tens of thousands of pounds on vitamin pills, the fact is that most doctors have never seen vitamin deficiency (such as scurvy, pellagra, or beriberi) in Britain.

In fact, if you make sure that you eat plenty of fruit, salads and green vegetables, and have average amounts of fish, meat, poultry, milk, butter or margarine, and bread, your chances of getting a vitamin deficiency disease in Britain are about the same as your chances of being eaten by a shark.

Indeed, the only common deficiency disorder of any sort in the UK is iron deficiency anaemia. This can hit you if you've spent many months on a diet low in iron-containing foods (*e.g.* eggs, meat, liver and fish), but most commonly it's due to heavy periods or some other cause of blood loss. But there is absolutely no need to supplement your diet with iron pills unless your doctor does a blood test, and says you're anaemic.

Protein, carbohydrate and fat

What about other important ingredients in the healthy diet? Among the most important is *protein*. This is the basic building material of the body, and it's contained in meats, offal, fish, cheese, milk, eggs and (to a lesser extent) in bread. However, once again there's little need for most people to worry about keeping their protein intake up, because in Britain protein deficiency is a great rarity.

The next ingredient in our diets is called *carbohydrate*. This word just means the sugars and starches—which are mainly contained in (of course) sugar itself, plus bread, potatoes, cakes, biscuits, sweets, puddings, rice and all the spaghetti-type foods. There is *no* risk whatever of anyone getting carbohydrate deficiency.

Indeed, children and young people eat far, far too much of carbohydrate foods, which look pretty or appeal to a sweet tooth but which contain very little apart from sugar. I'm talking about things like seaside rock, candy floss, sweets, ice lollies, biscuits, lollipops and sugary soft drinks, and, of course, chocolate-coated, yukky, sugar-laden confectionery!

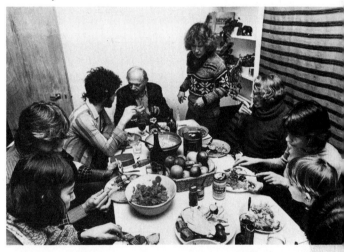

Finally, another major component of foodstuffs is the *fats*. They're contained in pastry, butter, margarine, cooking fat, and oils, fatty meat, and also milk and especially cream. Yet again, fat deficiency does not occur in the UK. And once again, it's generally felt among doctors that most of us eat far too much fat—especially animal fat.

This is not just because fat is *packed* full of calories and thus tends to make you fat too. It's because there is some evidence that over-consumption of animal fat may, at least in part, be responsible for the epidemic (and I do mean epidemic) of coronary disease that has hit Western man (and woman) so badly in the last 70 years. Many doctors do now make a conscious effort to keep down the amount of animal fat which they eat, for instance by spreading butter very thinly, or by switching to a SOFT vegetable margarine, or by going for grilled rather than fried food.

GOOD SLEEP AND RELAXATION

You can't be fit and healthy unless you have adequate relaxation and sleep. Research shows that if people don't get enough rest, their work suffers. Not only that, it's been shown that if they are under stress for long enough, there is a greatly increased risk of illness hitting them.

So, you must have enough sleep, and you must have enough time off. These days, there's a lot of talk (much of it quite justified) about how many downright lazy people there are around. But doctors see another side of things— for a lot of people who come into our surgeries are very far from lazy! These are men and women who flog away as hard as they can from dawn till dusk and way beyond, rarely taking a complete day off. This applies not only to people in paid employment, but to overworked housewives as well.

Doing this kind of thing is certain to lead to mental and physical exhaustion—and, unfortunately, it may lead to physical or mental breakdown too. If you've got a tendency to be a bit of a 'workaholic', then stand back and take a look at yourself. Ask yourself what you're trying to prove, and whether it wouldn't be better for both yourself and your family if you took more time off.

So, if you're overworking, then just bear in mind that the world won't come to an end if you have some time off. Indeed, you'll be more efficient at your work when you've had a rest.

People vary in the amount of relaxation they need, but it isn't usually a good idea to work more than about ten hours a day on a regular basis. If you have to work a really long spell of ten to fourteen hours, then you should try to only do a short shift on the next day.

How many days off a week do you need? Some people need two, some need only one—but nobody should have less than that. And—most important—you should try and get at least seven-to-eight-hours' sleep each night—preferably without the use of pills.

Bear in mind though that *older* people usually need a lot less sleep and can manage on five or six hours.

GOOD LOVE—AND GOOD SEX

I said in the last chapter that good health involves being happy—or, if you like, that good health incorporates good emotional health. An essential part of good emotional health is loving and being loved.

For the fact is that most people who are complete loners, with no wife or loving sexual partner, no family and no friends, are pretty miserable.

The great seventeenth-century poet, John Donne, is most often remembered for one single line—'No man is an island'.

And he was right: survival by yourself, without love and affection, is a grim and unhappy business.

In order to be loved, you need also to love. If you're a mature person, you know this already. But if you're young and haven't much experience of life, then try if you can to bear in mind that loving is a two-way business in which you have to be able to give as well as to receive. It can be a very difficult business too (not at all like the rosy picture so often presented in films and books and romantic magazines), but it's worth working at.

Sex

Then there's the sexual aspect of love. Although many people would disagree with me, I personally feel that a person is unlikely to be in the best of emotional health unless he or she is functioning properly where sex is concerned. Unfortunately, the results of sexual frustration are all too clear to doctors. If all this frustration disappeared overnight, then so too would many of the psychological problems that affect so many people. I strongly suspect that a good part of the enormous mountain of tranquillizers dished out in this country is really prescribed to people who are suffering from sheer sexual frustration.

So, a good sexual life is worth working at too. If you— like many people—have trouble in achieving a good sex life with your partner, then seek advice. Books are of some help (try the Family Planning Association Bookshop, 27–35 Mortimer Street, London, W1 or the Marriage Guidance Council Bookshop at Little Church Street, Rugby). If you need personal advice, then either talk to your doctor or go to a Family Planning Clinic, where they'll be pleased to chat with you. If you're young, then try the local Youth Advisory Clinic (which may be under your local authority's entry in the phone book) or else one of the Brook Advisory Centres (headquarters phone number 01-708 1234/1390).

All the above-mentioned people will also help you with safe contraception—which is a vital ingredient of almost any sexual relationship between a man and a woman. Since unwanted pregnancy is one of the real health problems of today, and as an unwanted pregnancy can now be almost completely avoided, you owe it to your partner and yourself not to run the risk of it.

Infection

The other major hazard of sex is infection—not just VD, but the minor genital infections which are also passed on by love-making. If you need confidential advice about any of these, you can obtain it from any of the agencies I've mentioned above.

But if you've risked VD (by having sex with someone

who may have been carrying an infection) or if you have symptoms 'down below' which you fear may be those of venereal disease, then the best course is usually to go straight to one of the network of over two hundred sexually-transmitted disease (STD) clinics which are in operation throughout the country. Just ring the nearest large hospital and ask the operator where the 'Special Clinic' can be found. Or go to your doctor. If you're a woman, bear in mind that VD usually produces *no* symptoms in its early stages—but big trouble later on.

GOOD SENSE ABOUT SMOKING AND DRINKING

Sorry to preach, but there is no doubt that smoking is one of the major health hazards in Britain today.

It causes far and away the most common cancer of men (and the third most common cancer of women), namely *lung* cancer. It kills many more people through heart and chest diseases, and leaves even more in rotten health in later life—coughing, wheezing and spluttering every winter.

And as far as fitness is concerned, it's more or less impossible to achieve top fitness if you're a smoker.

So why do people smoke? Partly because of the very addictive nature of nicotine—the drug which is contained in tobacco. There's a lot more to it than that, however, not least the social pressures which make it difficult for many young people to refuse an offered cigarette.

But the best way to avoid the health hazard of smoking is never to start. Once you're hooked (as most smokers are)

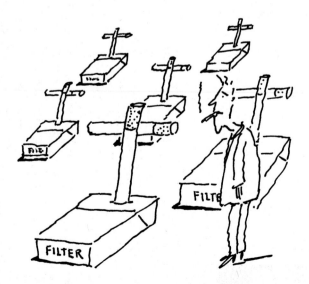

it's extremely difficult to give up. But it's worth trying very hard indeed.

Unfortunately, there are at present no drugs that will get you 'off the hook', though a new nicotine chewing gum may help a bit. I feel that the best hope is to go to an anti-smoking clinic, especially if they offer the 'group therapy' support of other people who are in the same boat. If you send a stamped, addressed envelope to Action on Smoking & Health, 27 Mortimer Street, London W1, they'll let you know the address of the nearest clinic to you.

Drinking

Alcohol isn't nearly as addictive as tobacco, so that most people are able to take it in moderation. But alcoholism is increasing, particularly among young people, which is rather worrying. Half a million British people are now thought to have a drinking problem.

Let's be clear that few doctors would dispute that small amounts of alcohol are quite harmless—and that drink can often be very useful in cheering people up and in helping to oil the social wheels of life. However, a considerable proportion of people do eventually get hooked on the stuff.

This isn't their fault. It's almost a natural tendency for many people to have a drink when they're upset or lonely or miserable. And when they've had enough booze on a regular basis for a long enough time, then the cells of their bodies become *dependent* on it.

Perhaps this wouldn't matter if it weren't for the fact that large quantities of alcohol eventually destroy the liver, and do great damage to the brain and other organs. That's why quite a lot of people die as a result of chronic alcoholism. Unfortunately, there's a lot of recent evidence that women are specifically at risk from this sort of damage.

As with smoking, don't get hooked in the first place. Modest amounts of alcohol normally won't cause you to become hooked, but it's surprisingly easy to get into trouble if a man exceeds about four pints of beer or a quarter bottle of spirits a day on a regular basis (and women's tolerance to alcohol is a good deal less.) That may not sound much—but it tots up to 28 pints a week, a fair amount!

Anyone who is taking a bottle of wine a day needs to watch his drinking carefully. A good rule is to have several alcohol-free days after an evening's drinking. The system has time to get rid of the products of the alcohol, helping to prevent the body's cells from getting dependent on the stuff.

And whatever you do, *don't drink and drive*. Any amount of booze in your bloodstream impairs your driving ability to some extent—and surprisingly modest amounts can put you in the mortuary.

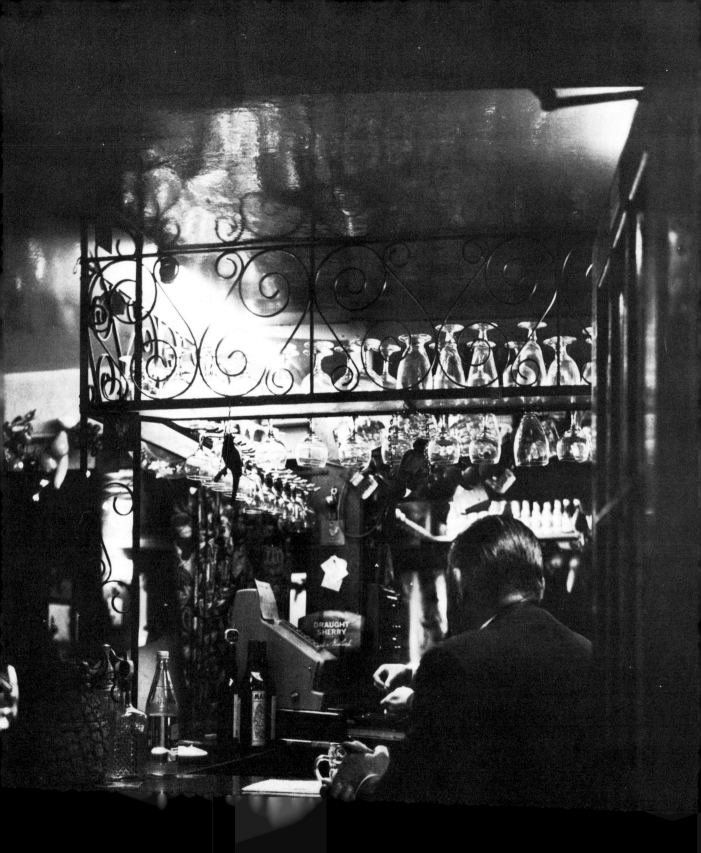

THE SEVEN AGES OF MAN (AND WOMAN)

The First Twelve Months

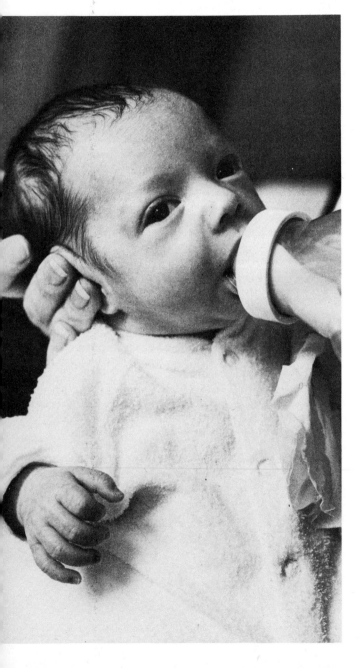

The first 12 months of life are the most hazardous of all (though someone once said that the *last* 12 often don't turn out too well either!)

In his famous story *The Vision of Mirzah*, the great writer Addison compared life to a long bridge or viaduct across which people were making their way. On the first few arches of the bridge (that is, in the first few weeks of life) there are many great gaping holes in the carriageway, through which young human beings fall into the abyss below.

But as one gets a little further along the bridge, the holes get fewer and fewer—and only towards the very end of it do they become more and more frequent again.

And Addison was right—life *is* like that. The first day of life is fairly dangerous (even in the 1980s), but the next week is far less so, and the risks to a baby's life steadily diminish over the course of his first year. In Britain today, the situation in a nutshell is this:

- Of 1,000 live-born babies, *993 survive the first week of life.*
- Of those 993 babies, *988 will make it to their first birthday.*

The figures are so much better than they used to be a generation or two ago—and so much better than those which apply in most other parts of the world—that I think that expectant mothers (and expectant fathers) can find them very reassuring indeed.

What can you do to make your child's chances of life and good health during his first year as good as possible?

I'd suggest the following points:

- Remember: care of your child starts as soon as you discover you're pregnant—or even when you're *trying* to get pregnant. Take care of yourself from then on—and you'll thereby take care of him too.
- Attend the best antenatal clinic you can find (yes, I must admit that one or two of them aren't too great!)
- From the time you know you're pregnant, try to cut out smoking—because it increases the risk of prematurity.
- Cut down on alcohol too—and most certainly avoid any real 'binges'—since there is now evidence that something called the 'foetal alcohol syndrome' (in plain words, baby damage due to booze) may exist.
- Don't take any drugs, pills or medicines unless it is ABSOLUTELY unavoidable. Prescribed vitamins are OK.
- If you're advised to rest because your blood pressure has gone up in pregnancy, then *rest*!
- As delivery time nears, take special care to attend your antenatal clinic sessions—and also any relaxation or National Childbirth Trust (NCT) classes if they are available.

LABOUR AND DELIVERY AND LACTATION

During labour and delivery, there's not a great deal which

you can do for your child, as matters are now largely in the hands of others. I am tempted to say that you should question the reasons for any obstetric intervention techniques—like induction of labour—but this isn't that easy when you're flat on your back and not feeling too bright.

But once labour's over and the babe safely delivered, then by far the best thing you can do for him is to insist on breastfeeding him.

There's not the least doubt, medically-speaking, that breastfed babies do better than babies fed on bottled milk (which is, after all, only modified cow juice). Furthermore, there's quite a lot of evidence that even *casual* bottle feeds given by the nurses "so as not to disturb mother" may be bad for the baby, by provoking an allergy to cow's milk protein. And you may have to struggle quite hard to PREVENT well-meaning nursing staff from shoving a bit of cow's milk down your unfortunate sprog.

ONCE YOU GET THE BABY HOME

When you take the baby home, you'll be guided by the Community Midwife and by the local Health Visitor.

Naturally, if the child seems unwell you may need to seek the advice of your GP too. Don't hesitate to do so if you're worried.

For I must admit that the first months with a new baby can be distinctly alarming—particularly if it's your *first* baby. (Life somehow seems to be a good deal calmer with second and subsequent babies!)

Lots of things happen during those first few months of life. Babies get colds; they get coughs; they vomit; sometimes they get diarrhoea; and very, very often they scream and scream—sometimes because of what seems to be a pain in the tummy, and sometimes for no apparent reason!

All I can say is that *most* such episodes DON'T turn out to be serious. But you should always ring your GP for advice in the following circumstances:

● If baby has a cough which makes it difficult to breathe.
● If he vomits up dark material (like coffee grounds).
● If he has 'projectile' vomiting—vomiting that shoots across the room.
● If he has diarrhoea that goes on for hours and hours, so that he's lost a lot of fluid.
● If he passes blood in his motions—this may look like red-currant jelly.
● If screaming attacks coupled with drawing up of the legs (as if in pain) go on for more than about five or six hours.
● If he has a fit (convulsion).
● If he develops a temperature of over 101°F (that's 38.3°C) taken under the armpit.

MILESTONES—AND IMMUNIZATIONS

Other things you need to know about during the first year of life are babies' 'milestones'.

What are milestones? They're the targets which the average baby should achieve at a given age. During the first year, I'd sum up the more important ones like this:

● At three months, a baby should be able to raise his head.
● Babies can usually sit upright without a hand to prop them up at about the age of six months, but some can't do this till nine months.
● Their first teeth *usually* appear at about this time (six to nine months).
● Crawling is very variable, but most babies start doing a spot of crawling around nine to 12 months.
● From 12 months (but up to 18 months in many cases), babies start learning to stand unaided—and then to walk.
● Talking is enormously variable, and a few children can use simple words like 'Mama' by 12 months. Few are like John Stuart Mill, who at the age of about one year hit his head and was asked by a lady if he was feeling 'an icky-bicky bit better.' He is said to have replied: 'I thank you, Madam: the agony has abated somewhat.'

Now, what about immunizations? Do for God's sake get these done. The immunization rate in the UK has dropped off dreadfully in recent years—all because of press publicity about the whooping cough jab.

If, after talking to your doctor and health visitor, you're still unhappy about the whooping cough injection, then don't let your child have it, but DO get the rest of the jabs done.

Government schedules change from time to time, but this is the current one. Your doctor or Child Health Clinic might wish to modify it if there are special circumstances—say, a tendency to convulsions—in your child's case.

First year immunization schedule (UK)

AGE	IMMUNIZATION	NOTES
3 months	First polio drops. First 'triple' jab—diphtheria, tetanus (lockjaw) and whooping cough.	Whooping cough can be left out if decided against.
$4\frac{1}{2}$ to 5 months	Second polio drops. Second 'triple' jab.	Ditto.
$8\frac{1}{2}$ to 11 months	Third polio drops. Third 'triple' jab.	Ditto.

Note: there are further immunizations AFTER the first 12 months. All will be revealed later in this chapter...

The Playschool Age

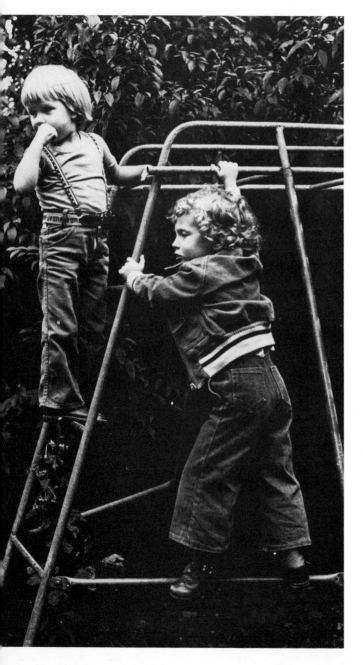

I'm taking the term 'the playschool age' to mean anything from one year to five years—though I must admit that not many kids go to playschool at one! However, one year olds can go to Day Nurseries—where they're exposed to the same (usually mild) health hazards that they'd be exposed to at playschool: namely, germs.

In fact, most of these germs aren't anything at all to worry about. Sure, they produce colds, coughs, perhaps the odd bout of tonsillitis, and sometimes a bit of a tummy upset. But your toddler *has* to meet them, *so that he can develop his own immunity to them.*

As to serious infections—he'll be pretty well protected against those if he's had the jabs and drops which I mentioned in the section on 'The First Twelve Months'. And he should continue this process of self-protection by having certain other immunizations during the pre-school years. These are:

AGE	IMMUNIZATION	NOTES
During second year	Measles jab.	More important than you probably think: measles can cause brain damage or even kill.
About five (*i.e.* school entry)	Booster polio drops. 'Double' vaccine booster—diphtheria and tetanus (lockjaw).	

What are the other hazards to your child in this age group? Well, by far the greatest is simply being killed in an accident, either:
● On the roads *or*
● In the home
ACCIDENTS ON THE ROADS. Terrifyingly, a recent survey showed that many parents thought it was quite OK for children under five years old to go out on the roads (even main roads!) by themselves. This is lunacy.

The biggest health danger to your child in the one-to-five age group is that a lorry will flatten him. Do *not* let him out in the street by himself, no matter how sensible he seems.
ACCIDENTS IN THE HOME. This is another very big health hazard in this age group, and many, many children die each year because of home accidents.

Here are some useful precautions which will help prevent such a disaster striking YOUR child:
● Lock away all pills, medicines and drugs. This includes things like aspirin and paracetamol (which can be killers),

and it includes medicines which the child is supposed to be on himself—it's all too easy for him to go and take a few more swigs of that funny stuff which Mummy likes him to have!

● Keep the youngster out of your kitchen if at all possible. (We found that having a stable door fitted to the kitchen was a wonderful way of doing this.)

If circumstances don't permit you to keep him out of the kitchen altogether, then for Heaven's sake get one of those cooker fittings which holds all saucepan handles safely in place—remember, a tipped-up saucepan can KILL a child.

● Keep all bottles of bleach or other caustic or poisonous household goods locked away out of the toddler's prying grasp. Above all, DON'T put such liquids in old lemonade bottles, or anything similar. The youngster will just assume —reasonably enough—that they *are* lemonade.

● If you have a fire, do not leave the child in the room near it unless there is a really good, strong fireguard which he cannot undo or knock over.

● Similarly, don't ever let a child of this age anywhere near a paraffin heater. Time and again, youngsters are attracted to these things—result: either a bad burn or (very often) the death of the entire family.

Development in the One-to-Five Age Group

This is a fascinating time of life, because your toddler is rapidly developing his own personality, learning to express himself—and learning how to try and manipulate YOU!

How fast should he develop? It's particularly important at this age to remember that youngsters develop *at their own pace.*

So, you shouldn't worry too much if the little boy or girl next door is talking a lot more than yours. As long as your toddler is beginning to make little sentences (like 'Sally want biscuit') by about the age of two, there's nothing to worry about.

Just remember too that *you yourself* should talk to your youngster as much as you can—because it's only in that way that he or she will be able to acquire the language.

One warning: if you're ever in the slightest doubt about whether your child can HEAR properly, then do get a proper hearing test arranged—either through your GP or through the Child Health Clinic. Many children are a little deaf, and failure to detect this at an early age can do great harm to a child's prospects of speaking well, as well as to his or her intellectual achievements.

How Fast Should the Toddler Grow?

The first 'chief' I ever worked for was a great paediatrician (he was paediatrician to Her Majesty the Queen, in fact), and he taught me that these were the expected weights of children during this period of their lives:

AGE	AVERAGE				
1	22 pounds	(approx. 10	kilos)		
2	28 ,,	(,,	12·7	,,	)
3	33 ,,	(,,	15	,,	)
4	37 ,,	(,,	16·8	,,	)
5	41 ,,	(,,	18·6	,,	)

More importantly, he also taught me that there was a great range of *variability*, and that, provided a child looked and felt well, there was no need to worry too much about minor deviations of a few pounds from the average.

But obviously, if your child looks 'skinny' and is far below the weights shown, then you *must* check with your doctor or Child Health Clinic.

More commonly in Britain these days, we find toddlers who are far, far above these weight figures—in other words, they're much too fat! Obesity is the most common nutritional disorder by far in this and other western countries, and unfortunately parents often don't realize that their child *is* obese—often thinking he's just a lovely, bonny, chubby boy or girl.

But by keeping him chubby and podgy, you may be laying up great trouble for him later in life. So once again, if your youngster's weight is way, way above those which I've quoted here, then check with your GP or Clinic that he's not too podgy. And if they think he's overweight, then take their advice about a sensible diet to get him into reasonable shape.

My old 'chief' also taught me about the *heights* which one could expect the average child to achieve in this age group. But once again, he made the point that there is tremendous individual variation. In particular, a child who comes of very tall or very short parents is likely to 'take after' Mum and Dad.

But as a general guide, here are the *average* heights in this age group:

AGE	HEIGHT			
1	29 inches	(approx.	73·5	cm)
2	33 inches	(,,	83·75	,,)
3	37 inches	(,,	94	,,)
4	40 inches	(,,	101·75	,,)
5	42 inches	(,,	106·75	,,)

Only if your toddler differs wildly from these norms without apparent reason need you check with your doctor.

The Younger Schoolchild
(5 to 12 years)

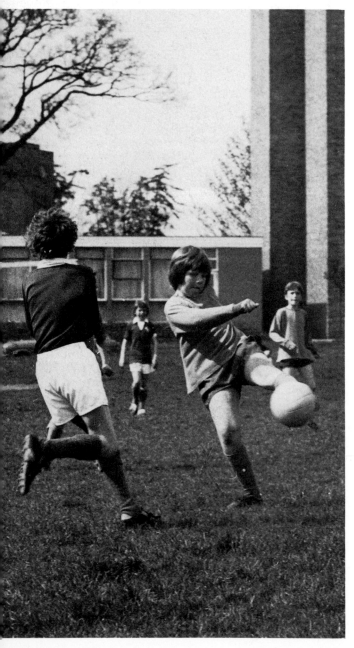

When your youngster goes to school, one of the most important things that happens to him is that he will be exposed to a *very* wide range of germs—considerably wider than he's encountered at playschool or day nursery.

The effect of this is very obvious. While some remarkably tough children get through those first few years at school with only a very occasional cough, the majority of kiddies are bound to have a considerable number of bouts of such infections as:

●Colds ●Earache ●Coughs ●Tonsillitis ●Tummy upsets (diarrhoea and vomiting).

But just as is the case with the germs which they meet in the earlier playschool period, *you just have to accept that your child will encounter these bugs.*

Furthermore, in many ways it's a GOOD thing, because the exposure to the germs gradually gives your child *immunity* to them. (I know it's easy for me to say that—but with all three of my children, I've been through that grotty period when the colds and coughs seem never-ending!)

In practice, though the years from five to eight or nine are often very, very trying, with lots and lots of colds and snuffles each winter, plus miserable bouts of earache and whatnot, the fact is that *at about nine most kids start developing a lot more resistance to these bugs.* Their health improves—and they start losing far less time from school.

DANGERS

Are there any particular health *dangers* in this age group? Once again, by far the biggest health risk is from accidents, both in the home and on the road.

Happily, kids become steadily less likely to have home accidents during this part of their lives—and, of course, most 11 or 12 year olds can quite safely be left in the house for an hour or two by themselves without doing anything crazy!

But because children tend to go out on the roads more and more as they get older, so the greatest risk to their lives by far becomes that of death on the roads.

In fact, therefore, the best things you can do to protect the life of your five-to-12 year old are these:

● Teach him the vital importance of the Green Cross Code.

● If you give him a bike, make sure that he is properly trained to use it and takes a Cycling Proficiency Test. Bear in mind that literally thousands of kids in this age group are badly injured on bikes in the course of a year.

Development in the Five-to-Twelve Age Group

Let's turn now to the question of how fast your five-to-12 year old should grow.

I'd repeat what I said in the section on the playschool period. There's tremendous individual variation, and you shouldn't worry at all if your youngster's weight differs by only a few pounds from the figures which I give here.

But once again, obesity is by far the greatest nutritional problem in this age group, and if your child's 'poundage' is far above what I quote here, then you really must see your GP and ask if the youngster needs a strict diet before things get hopelessly out of hand.

AGE	WEIGHT		
6	45 pounds	(approx. 20·4 kilos)	
7	49 pounds	(,, 22·3 ,,)	
8	55 pounds	(,, 25 ,,)	
9	61 pounds	(,, 27·7 ,,)	
10	67 pounds	(,, 30·5 ,,)	
11	73 pounds	(,, 33·2 ,,)	
12	79 pounds	(,, 35·9 ,,)	

What I've said about individual variation applies even more strongly to height. You shouldn't worry at all if your kids are some inches above or below the figures given in the following table—particularly if they're in the 11-to-12 age group, where a child's height increase depends very much on whether the 'growth spurt' of puberty is beginning to put in its appearance yet.

Only if your youngster is far below the figures quoted need you seek medical advice:

AGE	HEIGHT		
6	44 inches	(approx. 111·75 cm)	
7	46 inches	(,, 114·75 ,,)	
8	48 inches	(,, 122 ,,)	
9	50 inches	(,, 127 ,,)	
10	52 inches	(,, 132 ,,)	
11	54 inches	(,, 137 ,,)	
12	56 inches	(,, 142 ,,)	

IMMUNIZATIONS

I mentioned in the section on the pre-school period that kids need a booster injection of the 'double jab' (diphtheria and tetanus) when they're about five—together with a booster dose of polio drops. Fortunately, very few immunizations are needed in the years that follow.

In Britain at the moment, only *two* are required during this period. They are:

● Rubella (anti-German measles) vaccine for all girls aged 10 to 12.

● BCG (anti-TB) vaccine for all children aged 11 to 13 who have been shown by tests to be vulnerable to the disease (which means *most* kids).

Puberty and the Teenage Years

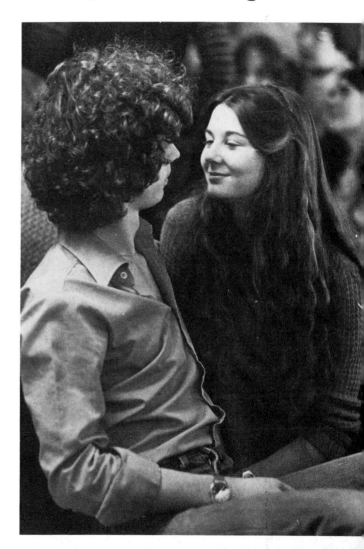

Lord, what a difficult period of life *this* is! For many children (and their parents!) it's a real nightmare—because of endless family conflicts, emotional problems, brushes with the Law, flirtations with drugs, experimentations with sex—and, of course, the excruciating problem of spots on the face!

But thank Heavens, it *is* possible to get through puberty and adolescence in a relatively tranquil fashion—provided that the child knows he or she is loved and wanted by his parents, and provided that he or she has been properly *prepared* for the changes of puberty. Sadly, even today far too many adolescent boys and girls are allowed to blunder through it all with no real help or prior teaching at all. (You'd be surprised at the number of girls who are told *nothing* about menstruation by their mothers until the day their first period arrives.)

Frankly, it's a wonder to me that so many kids turn out all right. But happily, most of them *do*. In fact, for the majority of young people, the problems of adolescence are fairly short-lived. But parents have to remember that skin troubles, difficulties with menstruation, worries about masturbation and other aspects of new-found sexuality—*all* may assume considerable importance in the adolescent's mind, and very understandably so too!

He or she should be helped to appreciate that, whatever the problem, it can be faced and overcome. The sensible, understanding parent who's always made a point of talking in a frank and friendly fashion with his/her child will find that this policy pays rich dividends as adolescence approaches. For the boy or girl who can *talk* about his or her difficulties is half-way to solving them. I'm afraid that it's in families where communication between parent and child has always been minimal that the greatest problems arise.

PREPARATION FOR ADOLESCENCE

Communication therefore has to start a great deal *earlier* than puberty. Preparation for adolescence, particularly in girls, has to start years ahead, partly because it's so difficult to predict the age at which sexual maturity will occur. (It may be any time from 10 to 16, and is sometimes actually outside this period! In general, it tends to occur slightly earlier in girls than in boys.)

Unfortunately, time and again parents put off telling their kids about sex until it's too late. The result may be that a terrified 14-year-old girl—probably miles from home —suddenly finds herself bleeding from the vagina and not knowing what a period is.

Or a frightened 15-year-old boy who knows next to nothing about sex (but who possesses sufficient male instincts to 'do it') may come home with VD. Or—as happens 5,000 times a year in Britain—a girl under the age of 16 may find that she is pregnant.

So, if the school doesn't teach this subject—and very few schools do it really adequately—make sure that you tell your own kids about the physical alterations that will take place in their bodies at puberty. And in due course (which to my mind

means when you see the first faint hints that puberty is about to happen) help them with advice about the powerful emotional changes that are going to overtake them soon.

Topics which all kids should know about by the age of 14 or so include the dangers of unwanted pregnancy, of VD, and of drugs. (Please don't say to yourself: 'There's no need for that with *my* child!' EVERY child is at risk these days.)

If you're in real difficulties and need a professional to counsel your youngster, remember that these days there are such things as the Brook Advisory Clinics (HQ telephone number: 01-708 1234) and also a small number of Local Authority Youth Advisory Centres (enquire at your town hall number about these). The doctors and counsellors there can be of enormous help in assisting your youngster through what can sometimes be one of the most difficult times of a person's life.

Puberty: From ages 11 to 17

The Younger Adult (From 20 Onwards)

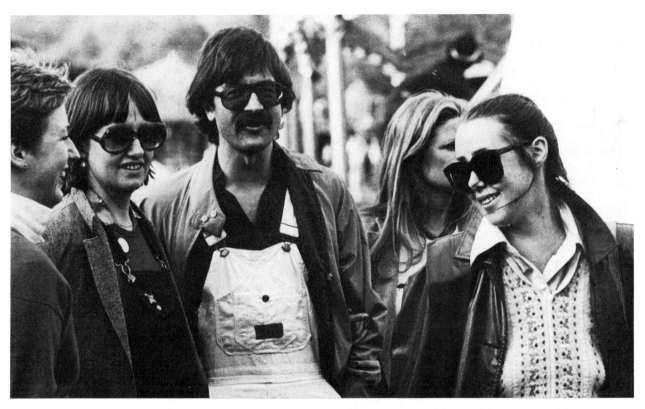

Happily, the period of youthful adulthood is the healthiest one of our lives.

True, there are dangers—the motor car or motor bike is still the number one killer. And there are still emotional storms of the kind experienced in the teenage years. So, depression, anxiety, and even hysteria are quite common—particularly among younger adults who are under a lot of strain because of exams, job interviews, unemployment—or problems with love affairs.

But by and large, the time from 20 to about 40 is the time when a person is *least* likely to have to go to a GP because of some illness. Young women are of course slightly different from young men in this period, due to the fact that they may have to seek medical help because of:

● Need for contraception
● Requests for termination of pregnancy (unfortunately)
● Gynaecological problems
● Childbirth

However, by and large, this is (or should be) a pretty healthy time of life. And it is also a time in which it's vital to establish good habits of the sort we've described in the earlier section of this book (A GUIDE TO A HEALTHY LIFE, page 13).

In brief, these healthy habits are:

● Not smoking
● Taking alcohol only in moderation
● Getting adequate exercise
● Eating a sensible diet
● Avoiding getting overweight
● Getting adequate sleep and rest
● Having a healthy (as opposed to a downright dangerous!) sex life.

It is important you establish these good habits in your twenties—because habits acquired at this period tend to stay with you for life.

The Middle Years

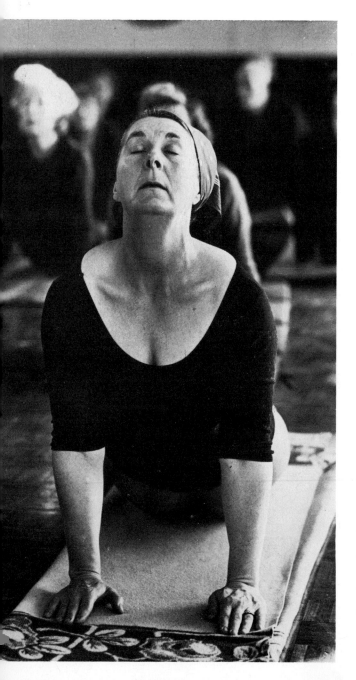

I don't know what *you* mean by the 'middle years'—but I think of them as the period from 40 to 60.

It's not the easiest time of life, either for men or for women. Both sexes have to face the fact that they are getting older, and that they may not have achieved all they wanted to in life.

Both sexes too may be worried by the fact that they are not as physically attractive as they once were—nor as physically fit. They usually have to visit the doctor more, as ailments like twinges of rheumatism and so on begin to creep up on them.

Then there is the undoubted deprivation seen in many middle-aged people when their families grow up and leave home—or when their partners die.

At work, the career-minded man or woman may find that younger men or women are coming along and beginning to 'threaten' them by being cleverer or quicker—or just by being cheeky or disrespectful! And for many career men and women these days, there's the sadness of finding yourself redundant—and perhaps, for a time, almost un-employable.

So all these pressures can create stress, anxiety and depression—all of which are very, very common at this age, particularly among women.

If *you* get symptoms of anxiety and/or depression, then beware of doing what so many people in 'mid-life crisis' do: that is, take solace in drink, cigarettes, overwork, and foolish sexual escapades.

It's far, far better to TALK to somebody—preferably your spouse, of course, but also close friends—and your family doctor. If he's good, he'll make time to listen to what you say, and to try to make helpful suggestions. Of course, the poor man's not a god or an oracle, so you can't expect him to re-fashion your life for you.

But a good GP can provide an awfully useful listening ear—or a shoulder to cry on. And when you really are suffering badly from depression, he can prescribe anti-depressant tablets that will help. I'm NOT talking about tranquillizers, incidentally—though these do have their place in the management of anxiety states. Antidepressants are completely different from tranquillizers, like Valium, because they are specifically designed to *reverse* the chemical changes in the brain which are so characteristic of depression.

THE MENOPAUSE

One of the great worries which people have in their middle years is the prospect of facing the menopause.

Let's get the blokes out of the way first. *There is no such thing as a menopause in men.* After all, 'menopause' actually means 'cessation of the periods'—and I need hardly remind you that men don't actually *have* periods! The various symptoms which people are all too ready to attribute to a 'male menopause' are actually due to such causes as psychological stress and overwork—*not* to hormonal changes. For men, unlike women, are very fortunate in that the output of their sex hormones falls only very, very slowly over a period of 20 to 30 years from the 40s onwards.

Women, however, are different in that their sex hormone output falls very rapidly indeed at the time of the menopause (average age 49 in Britain). This can result in very trying symptoms, which are described (together with treatment) in the A-to-Z section of 'Conditions' later in this book.

All I need stress here is that the menopause does NOT mean the end of your sex life, or of your physical attractiveness or womanly beauty. You may not even get any 'menopausal' symptoms—like hot flushes—but if you do, these can usually be treated fairly successfully nowadays with hormone replacement therapy.

KEEPING FIT

The other great thing to remember during these years is to KEEP FIT. Too many 'mediatric' (middle-aged) people let themselves get into terrible shape—becoming podgy, breathless, cigarette-dropping wrecks of their former selves. *Don't let it happen!*

Unlike the British, the Americans seem at last to have reversed the terrifying upward trend of heart disease in middle age—partly through following the sort of common-sense advice on diet and smoking and booze, which you'll find in the next section of this book, and probably, too, through *taking more exercise.*

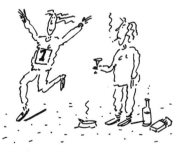

Personally, I thank Heaven for the jogging craze—for it has meant that many, many more middle-aged men and women are getting out and taking exercise, instead of sitting in front of that bloody TV!

Growing Older

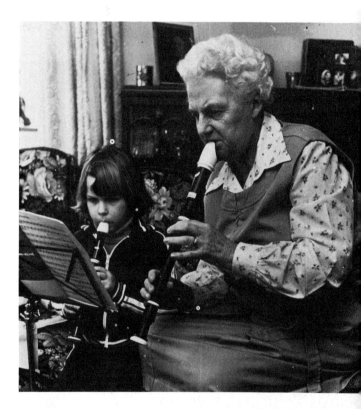

Shakespeare described the last of the seven ages of Man very cruelly:

> 'Last scene of all that ends this strange eventful history,
>   Is second childishness and mere oblivion,
>   *Sans* teeth, *sans* eyes, *sans* taste, *sans* everything...'

Well, there was probably a lot of truth to that in Shakespeare's day, when—so I understand from the Registrar General—most people only lived to about 40—and if you made it till 60, you were highly likely to be a physical wreck!

But these days things are very, very different. People are living a lot longer, and in general the *quality* of their life is much better too.

It would be dishonest of me to deny that *some* elderly people suffer very badly from physical ill-health, or from depression and dementia. But—and it's a very big BUT— the great majority of senior citizens can look forward to many happy years of interesting and fruitful retirement.

'Retirement' is possibly a key word—because it's important to make sure that when you reach that great watershed in your life, you don't just 'let yourself go'. It is absolutely *vital* at this stage of your lifespan to start looking around for new interests and hobbies, and to make as many friends as you can—and spend time enjoying yourself with them.

Don't sit at home—though the temptation to do so may be very great if you're feeling a bit tired or run down. People are particularly likely to become 'housebound' if they've recently lost a dearly-loved spouse, but this is just the time when it's important to get out: to the pub, to the local cricket club, to the Women's Institute, to the 'Pop-In Parlour' or wherever.

There are many good hobbies for older people to take up, which get them out of the house and keep them active—anything from golf, bowls and croquet to gardening and swimming and fishing.

And particularly satisfying are the activities which you can take up with your grandchildren (or with other children if you have no grandchildren of your own). There's a curious solace for many elderly people in seeing a new generation growing up, like spring after the winter.

Don't forget too that you should *exercise the mind* and keep it sharp. Memory may not be quite as good as it was, but that's no reason why you shouldn't make a point each day of 'stretching' your intellect in some way or another. I knew one 95-year-old retired pharmacist who embarked on an 'O' level course; and when I asked him why, he said, 'Because I've got to think of my future!'

YOUR DOCTOR

As the years advance, you'll almost certainly consult your doctor more than you used to. Indeed, he's paid a bit extra for the senior citizens on his list.

But it's NOT true, as so many people believe, that he is OBLIGED to visit all OAPs of over a certain age at regular intervals. So, if you've got a health problem, it's up to you to get in touch with him.

One word of warning. Many of the prescribed (and indeed unprescribed) pills and medicines consumed in this country are taken by senior citizens. And there's now a feeling among many doctors that a lot of OAPs take far too many drugs—*and that very often these drugs are doing them more harm than good.*

Again and again, I've visited old people's houses and flats and found the sideboards and mantlepieces and bedside cupboards absolutely *covered* in all sorts of tablets. Almost invariably, the patient hasn't been clear about what all the tablets are for, and how frequently they should take them. There's a special danger with sleeping pills, which can have the most disastrous effects on older people, sometimes even giving them hallucinations.

Families can assist here by helping to supervise tablets, and making sure that they're taken at the right time—and also in making sure that unwanted ones aren't left around the house where they can be taken by mistake!

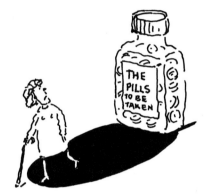

In fact, I think that families could play a very much greater part in the care of the older person in our society. Every GP is familiar with the situation where a family who hasn't seen Granny for six months pays a visit, finds her (not surprisingly) rather debilitated—and then rings up the doctor at 11 o'clock at night with an angry demand that 'something's got to be done!'.

When people say that, of course, they mean that they want the doctor to get Granny into a hospital right away—and off their hands!

Happily, many families *are* caring and thoughtful toward their older members. With the help of a loving family, with good friends and an understanding GP, today's senior citizen can look forward to a much happier retirement than has been possible at any previous time in history.

Let me close this section with Browning's lines about old age, which are a great deal more cheerful than Shakespeare's and—I think—often a lot more appropriate to today:

'Grow old along with me!
The best is yet to be,
The last of life, for which the first was made:
Our times are in His hand
Who saith "A whole I planned,
Youth shows but half; trust God: see all, nor be afraid!"'

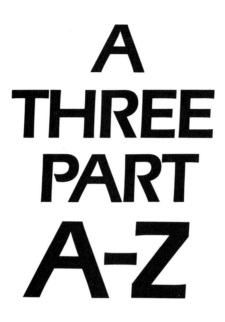

A-Z OF PARTS OF THE BODY

A

ADENOIDS

These are small pads of lymphatic tissue (rather like the tissue of the tonsils) found at the back of the cavity of the nose, just above the palate. The adenoids are usually relatively large in young children, and so may cause some degree of obstruction to the passage of air through the nasal cavity. A child who has this problem tends to snore a lot and to speak with a 'nasal' voice. Many such children grow out of this phase without any treatment. Others, however, have their adenoids removed (via the throat), usually at the same time as tonsillectomy is performed.

Considerable doubt has recently been cast on the value of widespread removal of the tonsils and adenoids (*see also* TONSILS AND TONSILLITIS under the A–Z of Conditions).

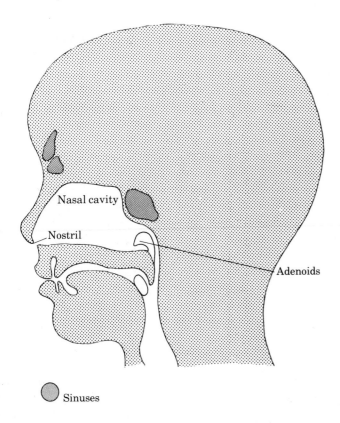

Nasal cavity

Nostril

Adenoids

Sinuses

ARTERIES

These are the tubes which carry blood *away* from the heart. (The tubes which carry it back again are the veins.) Unfortunately, they're very, very often affected by 'hardening of the arteries' in middle and later life.

This is a 'lay' term widely used to indicate degenerative disease of the arteries. (The posh medical word is arteriosclerosis.) One particular variety of this degeneration—known as atheroma—is the greatest killer in Western civilization. It narrows the calibre of various arteries, and thus diminishes the blood supply to vital organs such as the heart and the brain. The results are heart attacks ('coronaries') and strokes.

The causes of hardening of the arteries are not understood. At the present time, however, it appears that a person stands the best chance of avoiding it if: (a) he leads a physically active life with at least some exercise every day, and (b) he keeps his food intake and his weight down.

Foods that have been particularly incriminated in the development of atheroma are those rich in animal fats (butter, cooking fat, 'hard' margarine, milk and fatty meats), but some research has suggested that sugar may play a part. Smoking also very definitely contributes to the high incidence of diseases caused by atheroma. A vast amount of research is being done on the subject, and it is hoped that we will soon have some of the answers to this, one of the greatest problems facing medicine today.

B

BLADDER

This is the bag or 'sac', located just behind the pubic bone, in which urine collects. When a fair amount has collected, you feel the desire to pass water, as you may have noticed.

The one common disorder of the bladder is *cystitis* (*see* CYSTITIS in the A–Z of Conditions).

BOWELS

This is a rather vague term which basically means the lower intestines—the part of the intestine which leads down to the rectum and anus.

There are three bowel symptoms that demand immediate full investigation. *Widespread public knowledge of these simple facts would save many lives which are lost due to cancer.*

The three symptoms, which can sometimes indicate bowel growths, are:

(i) Bleeding from the bowel. While it is true that in young people this symptom is almost always caused by piles, in anyone over the age of about 35 the risk of cancer is appreciable. Examination by the doctor's finger will not confirm the presence of internal piles, so that it is essential to look inside the bowel with a special instrument: this usually entails going to a surgeon. (*See* PILES in the A–Z of Conditions.)

(ii) Black motions. This indicates bleeding from higher up the intestinal tract. The need for investigation is equally urgent, even though many patients turn out to have a benign condition, *e.g.* gastric or duodenal ulcer. (*See* **Peptic Ulcers** under ULCERS in the A–Z of Conditions.)

(*N.B.* Iron tablets and red wine also turn the motions black.)

(iii) Change in bowel habit. The unexplained onset of constipation or diarrhoea in a middle-aged or elderly person always raises the suspicion of serious bowel disease. If the doctor has any doubt whatever, he will order a barium enema X-ray or an examination of the bowel with a telescope-like device.

Chronic abdominal pain is also sometimes a symptom of serious bowel disease, and should be investigated.

Other common disorders of the bowel are dealt with under their various headings. (*See* CONSTIPATION; DIARRHOEA; DIVERTICULAR DISEASE; DYSENTERY; GASTRO-ENTERITIS; ULCERATIVE COLITIS in the A–Z of Conditions.)

BRAIN

The brain is, of course, not only the organ we think with, but the great 'nerve centre' of the body. Every movement we make is initiated by the 'motor' part of the brain, while every sensation which we perceive is actually registered on the 'sensory' part of the brain.

(*Note*: psychological disorders are dealt with separately, under the heading MENTAL ILLNESS in the A–Z of Conditions.)

The common physical disorders that effect the brain include injuries, vascular (blood vessel) conditions, degenerative diseases, infections and tumours.

Brain Injuries

These are very common after blows to the head. The belief, brought about by countless films and novels, that a human being can usually take a severe blow to the head with little or no effect (beyond a few minutes of unconsciousness) is dangerous nonsense!

Anyone who is struck a violent blow on the skull probably sustains some brain injury, however minor— which, I'm afraid, is why so many famous boxers become distinctly 'odd'. If slight confusion or even the shortest period of unconsciousness follows a blow to the head, the patient *must* go to hospital and have a full examination and an X-ray.

In many hospitals, it's the invariable practice to admit anyone who has been knocked out for a night's observation. Even so, a considerable number of patients with apparently trivial head injuries, and some of whom have not even been KO'd, still die each year because of undetectable brain damage.

The only answer to this problem is extreme caution. If you are struck on the head, always exercise considerable care during the next 24–48 hours. Don't take any alcohol, and see a doctor if you notice yourself becoming unusually drowsy or confused.

Vascular (Blood Vessel) Brain Disorders

These conditions are due to hardening of the arteries that supply the brain (*see* ARTERIES). They range in severity

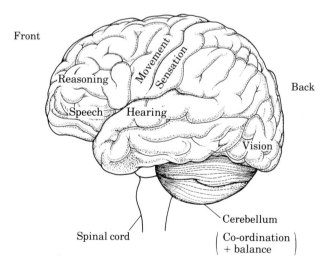

What happens where in the brain

from strokes (*see* STROKES in the A–Z of Conditions) to mild dizziness caused by transient impairment of the blood supply to the head. This latter symptom is extremely common in older people.

Degenerative Brain Disorders

There are several very rare types of brain degeneration which occur in middle age, but far more common is senile degeneration, which affects a percentage of people over the age of 70. Fortunately, many older people are quite untouched by this form of degeneration, and many others merely find that their memory and concentration are not quite what they used to be.

Sadly, some old people do however progress to *senile dementia*—a condition that is extremely trying for the relatives, but fortunately appears to inflict little suffering on the patient himself. Care in a long-stay geriatric hospital may be necessary.

However, it is being increasingly recognized that some old people diagnosed as suffering from incurable dementia due to brain degeneration do, in fact, have quite an element of depression (*see* DEPRESSION in the A–Z of Conditions), which is, of course, treatable.

Brain Infections

Though meningitis (*see* MENINGITIS in the A–Z of Conditions), or inflammation of the brain membranes, is quite common, infection of the brain itself is less frequent.

Encephalitis is a generalized brain inflammation, often due to a virus. *Cerebral abscess* is a collection of pus in the brain. It may follow ear or sinus infections, or a severe head injury. Treatment involves removal of the pus and administration of antibiotics.

Brain Tumours

A lot of people worry incessantly about brain tumours but they really aren't all that common. They may be primary or secondary. *Secondary* tumours are the result of spread from cancer elsewhere in the body. Unfortunately, they are mainly inoperable, but in fact often provide a merciful release to certain cancer patients.

Primary brain tumours are not very common, though an appreciable number are encountered in early childhood and in late life. Most adults who think they have brain tumours have no physical illness whatever; occasionally, people refuse to believe this and even kill themselves because they are convinced they have cancer.

Some primary tumours are benign, and even the malignant ones are often treatable. Symptoms include fits, par-

alysis of nerves (particularly those supplying the eyes, thus leading to squints), severe morning headaches over a period of weeks and persistent unexplained vomiting.

BREAST

The human breast is of course one of the most wonderful organs in nature. Not only is it immensely attractive (an important factor in what Darwin called the 'sexual selection' of the human race), but also it's a quite brilliantly-designed source of food for the human baby.

Disorders of the Breast

The most important breast disorder by far is cancer, and the most important point to bear in mind in regard to this condition is this: *every woman over the age of 25 should practise regular self-examination of the breasts.*

An examination once a month should be sufficient. Feel all over the breast tissue, using the flat of the hands. If there is any lump present, see your doctor within 24 hours.

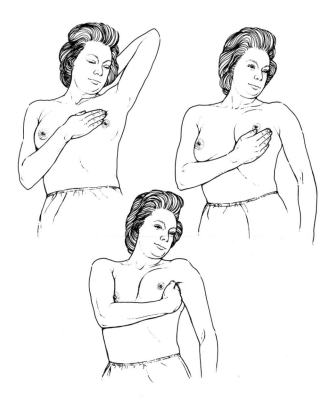

The correct way to check for lumps in the breast

What happens if you consult your doctor because you think you have found a lump? He will, of course, examine you himself to confirm that one is present. (Some women understandably mistake a slight thickening of the breast tissue for a lump.) Having assessed the swelling, he will arrange an urgent referral to a surgeon, who will usually perform a minor diagnostic operation on the breast within a few days.

This operation involves taking away a tiny portion of the lump for examination under the microscope. This procedure will show whether cancer is present. If it is, treatment will be started immediately.

The treatment of early breast cancer is nowadays fairly successful. This isn't the place to discuss the merits of the various methods of surgery and radiotherapy. Suffice it to say that the woman who has gone to her doctor *immediately* she has discovered a lump stands an excellent chance of living to a healthy old age.

Women tend, quite naturally, to be very frightened of the idea of losing a breast, but the courage that most women show in the face of this disease is quite remarkable.

N.B. Although breast cancer almost always makes the appearance in the form of a lump, it can sometimes cause other symptoms instead. The most common are *(i)* bleeding from the nipple, *(ii)* recent (as opposed to lifelong) in-turning of the nipple, *(iii)* puckering of the skin of the breast, *(iv)* a raw, weepy area developing on the nipple.

Other Breast Conditions

SWELLINGS. There are many benign causes of lumps in the breast but, as explained above, tissue from all such lumps must be examined under the microscope within a matter of days. Removing a benign lump is a simple matter, and no further trouble need be anticipated after the operation.

OVER- AND UNDER-SIZED BREASTS. Many women are understandably dissatisfied with the size of their breasts. Where the bosom is very big or small, plastic surgery can sometimes help. Hormone creams should not be used, as they are dangerous. Many proprietary 'bust-developing' preparations are completely useless. The most popular 'bust-developer' in the world is, in fact, a simple exercise, the object of which is to develop the muscles that lie behind the breast. It has at least the merit of being harmless!

MASTITIS. This means inflammation of the breasts. Most types of mastitis are fairly trivial, and respond moderately well to simple measures, such as wearing a better-fitting bra. Infective mastitis, however, will need antibiotic treatment and may progress to the stage of a breast abscess (*see* below).

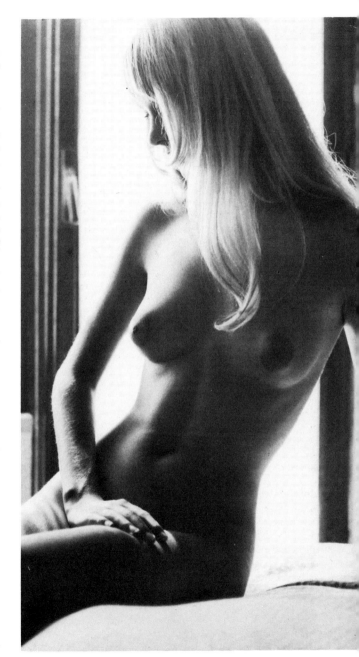

Not only lovely to look at, a woman's breasts also serve a supremely useful purpose.

BREAST ABSCESS. This is a common condition, at least during lactation. A painful swelling develops in the affected breast, and the overlying skin becomes reddened. Incision to drain off the pus relieves the pain and, together with the administration of antibiotics, leads to rapid healing.

C

CERVIX

The cervix is the neck of the womb—the soft cone of tissue that can be felt projecting down into the top of the vagina.

Cancer of the Cervix

Far and away the most serious disorder of the cervix is cancer. This condition causes about 2,000 deaths a year in Britain—mainly in women aged 45–60, but with a few deaths now occurring in the under 30s. The tragedy is that virtually all these deaths could be prevented by public education about cancer, the reason being that early cancer of the cervix is almost always curable. *Don't be afraid of using the Health Service to help you.*

SCREENING. Cancer of the cervix can be detected before it produces symptoms by means of the 'Pap' smear technique. I can't stress too strongly that every woman (especially every mother) over the age of about 23 should have this test performed at the intervals suggested by her doctor, *regardless of how well she feels.* Your doctor or local Family Planning Clinic will tell you how to have it carried out. Some doctors now want to do the test on teenagers, but it's doubtful if this would be cost-effective, as the peak age for deaths is 50 to 60.

SYMPTOMS. Any woman (especially who has not recently had a satisfactory 'Pap' smear) should watch out for the following symptoms:
● Bleeding after intercourse.
● Bleeding between periods.
● Unexplained pain in the pelvic region, including pain on intercourse.

See your doctor within a few days, even if bleeding is confined to a few spots of blood or a faint brownish discharge. He will do an internal examination, look at the cervix and probably refer you to a gynaecologist—unless there's some obvious reason, such as the contraceptive Pill you're taking doesn't suit you.

Other Cervix Disorders

CERVICITIS. A form of inflammation which is quite common. The principal symptom is discharge. Simple local treatment as an outpatient is usually curative.

CERVICAL EROSION. This is a trivial complaint which can produce slight vaginal bleeding and discharge. It commonly occurs after childbirth. Treatment is hardly ever necessary unless an erosion produces pain on intercourse or a trying amount of discharge. In these cases, 'cautery' (with a chemical or hot probe) will give a rapid and virtually painless cure.

POLYPS OF THE CERVIX. These occur at all ages, and cause discharge and slight bleeding. Removal is very easy.

E

EAR

The ear is the organ for hearing, and for balance. For individual ear disorders, look in the A–Z of Conditions.

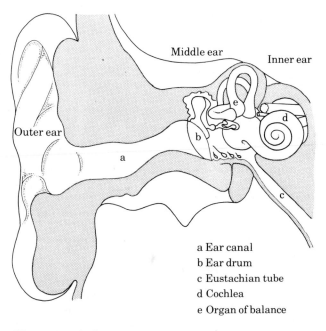

a Ear canal
b Ear drum
c Eustachian tube
d Cochlea
e Organ of balance

What is where in the ear

Hearing

Noise produces air waves, and these enter the ear, strike the ear-drum, and make it vibrate. The resulting vibration is transmitted by three small bones to the 'nerve apparatus' of the ear, which is connected to the part of the brain where hearing is registered.

Balance

To a large extent, the balance of the body is dependent on the parts of the inner ear called the 'semi-circular canals'. These contain fluid which swirls around when we move our head or turn around. Nerves connected with these canals relay information about the position of the body in space to the balance co-ordination centres of the brain.

G

GALL BLADDER

The gall bladder is a pear-shaped sac which lies in the upper right-hand part of the abdomen, just below the liver. The liver produces bile (which helps in the process of digestion of foods), and this bile is concentrated and stored in the gall bladder.

Disorders of this organ are common and are usually associated with gall stones. Gall stones are traditionally said to be liable to develop in patients who are 'fair, fat, female, fertile, flatulent and fifty'. They can, however, occur in any age group, and are quite frequently seen in males as well as females.

The symptoms of gall stones vary. Often, they cause no symptoms at all, and are only noticed on a routine X-ray, or during an operation for some other condition. But chronic upper abdominal pain is common; this often occurs a little to the right of the mid-line, just under the lower margin of the ribs.

If a small stone becomes jammed in the neck of the gall bladder or in the cystic duct (the tube which carries the bile away from the organ), the result is *gall stone colic*. This is an excruciating pain which runs from the area mentioned above to the region of the right shoulder blade. The attack is usually accompanied by retching and vomiting. Applying a hot water bottle to the tummy will give some relief until the doctor arrives.

Gall stone jaundice is due to a stone becoming jammed

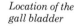

Location of the gall bladder

slightly lower down the biliary tract, so that bile pigment cannot get out of the liver and overflows into the blood. The patient goes yellow and often experiences intense itching. His urine becomes dark and the motions become putty coloured.

Investigation and Treatment

An ordinary X-ray of the abdomen may sometimes be helpful since gall stones containing calcium will show up on it, but many patients need to have special X-rays in which a dye is either taken by mouth (an oral cholecystogram) or given by injection (an intravenous cholangiogram). It may also be necessary to operate, in order to carry out even more sophisticated X-rays, in which dye is injected directly into the bile passages. A new technique now enables this to be done without surgery.

Treatment of gall bladder disease is a complex business. Very often (*e.g.* in acute cholecystitis) purely 'medical' methods are adequate. Many patients with gall bladder disorders require surgery, however, and most of these undergo the operation of cholecystectomy, or removal of the gall bladder. The results of this procedure are usually very good.

Two new drugs will dissolve certain kinds of gall stone— but only certain kinds! If they fulfil their present early promise then they'll make much gall bladder surgery unnecessary in the future.

K

KIDNEYS

The two kidneys are situated at the back of the abdominal cavity, just under where the lowest ribs meet the spine. They have two functions: *(i)* to filter poisonous waste products out of the blood for excretion in the urine; and *(ii)* to maintain the vital chemical balance of the body. The kidneys are therefore essential to life (though one can be safely removed if necessary, since the other will take over its work). Where the function of both is seriously impaired, regular treatment with an artificial kidney machine may sometimes be life-saving. A kidney transplant can often provide a permanent cure.

There are many rare disorders of the kidney, and I'm only going to deal with a few of the commonest ones here. (*And see also* BLOOD PRESSURE under A–Z of Conditions.)

Nephritis

This means inflammation of the kidney. The term is applied to a number of separate conditions, and unfortunately doctors differ considerably in the way they classify them.
ACUTE NEPHRITIS. This is a disorder in which loss of kidney function causes fluid retention, and hence puffiness of the face. The urine often contains blood. The patient, who is usually a child, may have had a throat infection about a fortnight before the attack. Most children make a fairly rapid recovery.
NEPHROTIC SYNDROME. A state characterized by massive swelling of the face and the whole body. The illness is likely

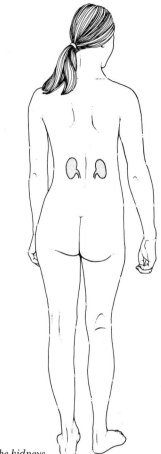

Location of the kidneys

to be much more prolonged than is the case with acute nephritis, and complex investigations will be necessary.
CHRONIC NEPHRITIS. A long-standing kidney inflammation which is the end result of a number of different kidney disorders. The disease usually runs an intermittent course over many years, and careful supervision at a specialist clinic is desirable.

Kidney Infections

These are potentially dangerous conditions which should be treated with respect and always investigated thoroughly. Some of them start with a bout of cystitis (*see* CYSTITIS in the A–Z of Conditions) which has been ignored.
PYELITIS AND PYELONEPHRITIS. These are virtually the

same condition and are both dealt with under the heading PYELITIS in the A–Z of Conditions.

TB OF THE KIDNEY. Much less common than it used to be, this condition is treated by anti-tuberculous drugs and sometimes by surgery.

Kidney Stones

These are quite common and may sometimes be secondary to some other disorder such as malfunction of the parathyroid glands. Small stones may pass down into the ureter (the narrow tube that carries urine down to the bladder) and become jammed. This causes the intense pain called renal colic. Unless stones are passed out in the urine, they usually have to be removed surgically.

L

LIVER
(See also GALL BLADDER, *above,* and CIRRHOSIS and JAUNDICE in the A–Z of Conditions.)

The liver is a large organ (in fact the single *largest* organ in the body) located in the top right hand corner of the tummy, where it's shielded by the lower ribs. From the health point of view, the most important thing about it is that it's easily damaged by certain chemical agents—especially alcohol. The liver has many functions, the most important of which are to break down drugs and other potentially harmful agents (including alcohol) to make bile—which helps digest the fat we eat—and to act as a reserve store for carbohydrates.

LUNGS
(See also ASTHMA, BRONCHIECTASIS, BRONCHIOLITIS, BRONCHITIS, COUGH, EMPHYSEMA, PLEURISY, PNEUMOCONIOSIS, PNEUMONIA, PNEUMOTHORAX, PULMONARY EMBOLISM, and TUBERCULOSIS in the A–Z of Conditions.)

The lungs are two large 'sacs' which become filled with air as we breathe in. One lung is in the right side of the chest, the other in the left side. The *function* of each lung is to extract oxygen from the air and transfer it to the blood stream. On the other hand, 'waste' gas carbon dioxide passes out of the bloodstream in the lungs, and is exhaled in the air we breathe out.

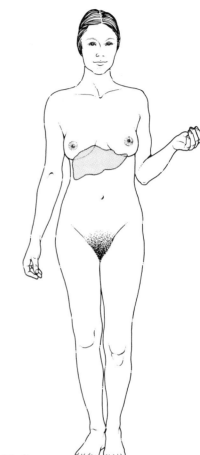

Location of the liver

P

PROSTATE GLAND

This is a gland about the size of a large chestnut which lies at the neck of the male bladder. There is no exactly corresponding structure in women, though recent research suggests that women have a similar glandular region which is highly sexually responsive. The prostate gland produces a liquid which forms part of the seminal fluid.

The urinary passage goes right through the prostate, and the unfortunate consequence of this is that enlargement of the gland will block the flow of urine from the bladder, either completely or partially.

The cause of the enlargement of the prostate is not known, but, like greying of the hair, and stiffness of the joints, it's probably just another consequence of ageing. It doesn't seem to affect sexual function at all.

The patient with an enlarged prostate usually notices that he has some difficulty in producing a good stream of urine, and that sometimes it may be very difficult to 'get started', particularly when the bladder is full. Most patients are obliged to get up once or twice at night to pass water.

There is also a risk of *acute retention* developing; in this condition, no urine can get out of the bladder at all and prompt treatment is necessary. The subject is discussed fully under the heading RETENTION OF URINE in the A–Z of Conditions.

Treatment of an Enlarged Prostate

GENERAL. Many mild cases of prostatic enlargement can be kept in check by simple medical means. If you have a moderately enlarged prostate, you should avoid drinking large quantities of fluid, particularly alcohol, tea and coffee, all of which tend to increase the flow of urine. (These drinks are quite all right in moderation, however.)

Make sure you empty your bladder regularly—say, every one to two hours, and especially before setting off on long journeys. The worst possible thing to do, for instance, would be to have several pints of beer before a long, unbroken car ride home on a cold night—this would be inviting an attack of acute retention.

Another important point to remember is that prostate sufferers are particularly liable to inflammation of the bladder or cystitis (*see* CYSTITIS in the A–Z of Conditions), and, in fact, any kind of urinary infection. So, if you get pain and discomfort on passing water, see your doctor as soon as possible, so that he can send a carefully collected specimen of urine to the lab for culture.

SURGICAL. When prostate trouble gets too bad, surgery is essential. About one prostate patient in four eventually needs an operation. It's now often possible to carry out what's called a TUR (or transurethral resection), which simply involves pushing a slim telescope with a cutting device up the urinary passage, and nibbling away bits of the prostate so as to make the passage wider. But the surgeon may operate to remove the whole prostate gland.

This procedure (prostatectomy, as it's called) at one time used to be very dangerous, and very distressing for the patient. Nowadays, it's a straightforward and safe business, though the few days after the operation are not usually much fun.

Most patients do very well, however, and are out of hospital within about two weeks. A month or so of convalescence will be required. Urinary control should usually be regained shortly after the operation.

There should usually be no serious interference with sexual function, and some men, because of improved general good health, actually enjoy happier marital relations after the operation. Seminal fluid will no longer be produced at orgasm, which means that the man will probably be unable to have further children. Since most patients are at least in their late fifties, and have long completed their families, this is not usually of any consequence.

Cancer of the Prostate

When a patient who has symptoms of prostate trouble seeks medical advice, the doctor will always do a rectal examination, since this enables him to feel the size, shape and texture of the gland with his finger. If the gland feels craggy and hard, cancer may be present, but I must stress that cancer is *rare* compared with ordinary benign enlargement of the gland.

Cure of prostatic cancer can be achieved by complete removal of the gland. Some patients are treated with hormones.

Many doctors, especially in the US, feel that all males over the age of 45 should have a yearly rectal examination to detect both benign and malignant disease of the prostate, as well as disorders of the rectum itself. Lives could probably be saved by this sort of universal screening, but the costs would be considerable.

SPLEEN

The spleen is a blood-forming organ that lies high up in the left-hand side of the abdomen, under the protection of the lower ribs. A heavy blow in this region may rupture the spleen and cause severe or even fatal bleeding. Unfortunately, the patient may seem and feel perfectly well for a period of several hours while the haemorrhage is going on. If you sustain a severe blow to the abdomen or chest, for instance in a road accident, it's always best to go to hospital for a check-up, no matter how well you may feel.

T

THYROID GLAND

The thyroid gland, situated at the front of the neck, is subject to various disorders. It's basic function is to produce *thyroid* hormone—a sort of 'get up and go' hormone which stimulates much of the rest of the body into activity.

Goitre

A goitre is simply a swelling of the thyroid gland. A slight degree of swelling is very common in women at specific times—at puberty, at the menopause, during pregnancy, and sometimes during periods. These very slight enlargements, which scarcely deserve the name 'goitre', don't usually need any treatment apart from an occasional check by the doctor.

Other goitres may be caused by lack of iodine in the diet, though this is rare in developed countries nowadays.

Goitre may also be due to benign thyroid growths, and sometimes malignancy. It's far more frequent, however, for a thyroid swelling to be due to over-activity of the gland (see below).

Overactivity of the Thyroid

Hyperthyroidism, thyrotoxicosis, and Grave's disease, are all medical terms which mean the same thing—overactivity of the thyroid gland. This condition is common, particularly in women. The patient usually has a moderate goitre. She complains of losing weight (despite an increased appetite), irritability, nervousness, and inability to tolerate warm weather. Her face is usually thin and her eyes are prominent and staring.

Hyperthyroidism can be treated in three ways: by anti-thyroid drugs, by surgical removal of most of the gland (thyroidectomy), or by use of a radio-active preparation.

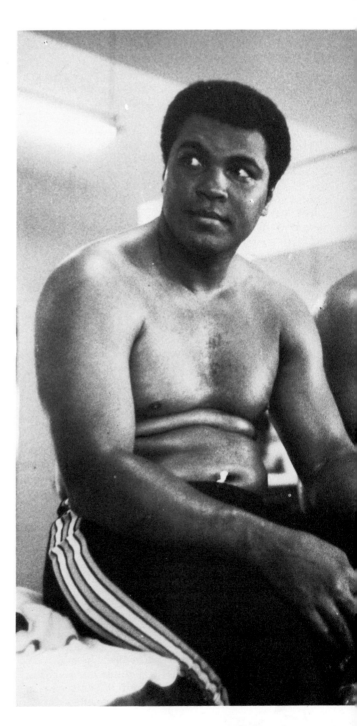

Mohammed Ali was indeed 'The Greatest' when he fought Joe Bugner. It was widely reported that he tried to lose weight by taking thyroid tablets—but these should never be used for slimming.

All three methods give very good results, though the symptom of staring eyes is sometimes difficult to treat. The late, great Marty Feldman had this problem.

The use of radio-activity is not advisable in people of child-bearing age, and these patients are normally treated either by surgery or by anti-thyroid drugs.

Underactivity of the Thyroid

INFANTS. Babies who suffer from underactivity of the thyroid are liable to become cretins unless the condition is diagnosed early on, so that treatment with a thyroid hormone can be started. Adult cretins are mentally deficient and stunted, but fortunately this sad condition is not often seen these days because, in developed countries, most babies are given frequent health checks in the early months of life. Though cretinism is not normally detectable at birth, it can usually be diagnosed by about the age of two months. Treatment started then will ensure normal development.

ADULTS. Underactivity of the thyroid starting in adult life is called myxoedema. The features are essentially the opposite of those of overactivity of the gland (see above). Thus, the patient puts on weight (despite having little appetite). He gets slow and lethargic, and detests cold weather. The face becomes bloated in appearance, and the skin and hair coarsen. There may be a smallish goitre.

Treatment of myxoedema with thyroid hormone preparations dramatically reverses these changes, and restores the patient to completely normal health.

VAGINA

The vagina, or 'front passage' as it's often quaintly called, is the wide, spacious, moist and well-cushioned channel which leads from the exterior up to the neck of the womb.

The word 'vagina' is Latin for 'sheath', and the reason for the name is of course the fact that the vagina provides an ideal 'sheath' for the penis, I'm glad to say.

There are many disorders of the vagina, and some of them can be extremely distressing for a woman. In this particular sphere, far too many patients suffer in silence. If you have some sort of vaginal trouble, the golden rule is to go and see your doctor before things get any worse. Don't delay because of embarrassment. The doctor will examine you and, if necessary, order lab tests or send you to

see a gynaecologist. Family planning clinics provide another source of advice.

Vaginal Bleeding

Any type of vaginal bleeding other than the blood loss associated with completely regular periods needs assessment by a doctor.

BLEEDING DURING PERIODS (MENSTRUATION). Heavy menstrual blood loss ('flooding') and irregular menstruation can readily cause anaemia, and should be treated as soon as possible. (*See also* PERIOD PROBLEMS in the A–Z of Conditions.)

BLEEDING BETWEEN PERIODS. Intermenstrual bleeding or bleeding after intercourse (even if it's only 'spotting' on the underclothes) may be a serious symptom. A full gynaecological examination is advisable. See your doctor within two or three days. But 'spotting' can also be due to an inappropriate brand of Pill.

BLEEDING AFTER THE MENOPAUSE. This too may be a serious symptom and needs immediate gynaecological assessment. Again, consult your doctor at the earliest possible date. (*See also* MENOPAUSE in the A–Z of Conditions.)

BLEEDING IN PREGNANCY. In early pregnancy (up to five months), bleeding is usually due to a threatened or actual miscarriage (abortion). See the warning note, under MISCARRIAGE in the A–Z of Conditions. In late pregnancy, bleeding may be due to various causes. (*See* Disorders of Pregnancy, under PREGNANCY in the A–Z of Conditions.)

Vaginal Irritation and Discharge

IRRITATION. Vaginal irritation usually occurs together with irritation of the vulva, and is dealt with under the heading PRURITUS in the A–Z of Conditions. Irritation often occurs in combination with discharge (*see below*).

DISCHARGE. One of the commonest of all symptoms, and one that causes a great deal of worry—often unnecessary worry, at that.

It's important to stress that from puberty onwards, a certain amount of vaginal secretion is completely normal. A lot of teenage girls don't realize this. Because they're often embarrassed about consulting their own doctors, they deluge newspaper and magazine advice columns with letters about this problem.

The vaginal fluid should be thin and reasonably clear; it has a natural aroma, the presence of which does not indicate a need for the use of douches or vaginal deodorants. The rate of secretion of the fluid varies from time to time and increases markedly when sexually aroused.

So when does a discharge need medical attention? Basically, if it's thick, if it's yellow, green, brown or red, if it's irritant or associated with soreness or pain, or if it smells offensive.

Causes of discharge include disorders of the cervix (neck of the womb), and particularly cervicitis, cervical erosion and cervical polyps (*see* CERVIX). Other common causes are infection by thrush (*see* THRUSH in the A–Z of Conditions) and by the trichomonas parasite (*see* TRICHO-MONAS INFECTION OF THE VAGINA in the A–Z of Conditions).

It's worth knowing that lately we've discovered that certain 'new germs' can cause vaginal discharge. A very common one is called Gardnerella vaginalis, which causes a greyish discharge with an embarrassing smell. It's treatable with Flagyl tablets. Also, never forget that a forgotten tampon can be a cause of vaginal discharge.

If you have one of the types of discharge outlined above, see your doctor. He will examine you and may send swabs to the lab for examination. If necessary, he will arrange an appointment with a gynaecologist.

Most types of vaginal discharge and irritation respond promptly to adequate treatment, though recurrences may occur in some cases. In view of the recent emergence of 'new' vaginal infections (like Herpes), if in doubt don't hesitate to go to a 'special', or 'genito-urinary', clinic.

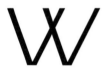

WOMB

The womb, or uterus, is a pear-shaped organ. It's about the size of an average-weight pear too—and if you imagine the womb as a nice Conference pear standing on its tip in the lower part of your body, you won't be far wrong! The 'tip' represents the CERVIX (see page 34)—the neck of the womb which projects down into the vagina.

There are many disorders of the womb. They include endometriosis, fibroids and metropathia (*see* ENDOMETRI-OSIS, FIBROIDS and METROPATHIA in the A–Z of Conditions), cancer of the womb, and prolapse of the womb (*see below*).

Cancer

Cancer is NOT all that common, so please don't be terrified by this section! Cancer can occur either in the body of the womb or in the neck, or cervix. I've dealt with cancer of the cervix under CERVIX.

Cancer of the *body* of the womb reaches a peak among women in the age group 40–55, but may occur outside these limits. There's now some evidence that poorly supervised hormone replacement therapy (HRT) may provoke it. It's also most likely to be seen among those who have never borne children. The chief symptoms are either bleeding after the menopause or irregular bleeding at or before the menopause. The bleeding may be in the form of a blood-stained or brown discharge, which may later become offensive.

Cure can be achieved if the disease is caught early. If you have these symptoms, you need a full gynaecological examination urgently. If this reveals no straightforward and harmless cause for the bleeding or discharge, you'll probably have a 'D and C', or scrape of the womb. If this shows cancer, you'll usually have a hysterectomy (*see* HYS-TERECTOMY in the A–Z of Conditions).

Most women wait four to seven months after the onset of symptoms before going to their doctors. Make sure *you* don't do the same.

Prolapse of the Womb

Almost any woman who has had a baby will have some looseness of the pelvic tissues afterwards, and this tends to increase with subsequent children.

In many women, the result is that in middle life the womb tends to sag downwards into the vagina. Often, the vaginal walls will sag too, and this may cause problems with the bladder, which lies just in front of the vagina.

If you have a prolapse of the womb or the vaginal walls you may notice a feeling of weakness or 'bearing down'. You may keep passing water without meaning to. If the prolapse is severe, the cervix, or neck of the womb, may appear at the opening of the vagina.

The best treatment of prolapse is with surgery. Usually, the surgeon does a neat repair operation through the vaginal opening. There are no scars to see, and the general tightening up of tissues usually has a beneficial effect on sexual relations. Further pregnancy is not always a good idea, however, and your gynaecologist will advise you on this point.

In severe cases of prolapse, hysterectomy is often necessary (*see* HYSTERECTOMY in the A–Z of Conditions).

Occasionally, a patient with prolapse is not fit enough to undergo surgery. In these cases only, a supporting 'pessary' can be placed in the vagina. Very, very mild prolapse can be improved by exercise.

A-Z OF CONDITIONS AND DISEASES

A

ABDOMINAL PAIN

Where tummy pain is concerned, readers shouldn't be tempted into self-diagnosis or self-treatment. If in doubt about any abdominal pain, *consult your doctor*. Do not take aspirin or laxatives, both of which may make abdominal disorders worse. (Remember that most proprietary pain-killers—except paracetamol—contain aspirin.)

Chronic (*i.e.* longstanding) Abdominal Pain

This is a common symptom, and one which middle-aged and elderly people may ignore to their cost.

Any pain or discomfort, however slight, that has per-sisted for over a week or more, should be fully investigated. Your doctor will examine you carefully, often carrying out a rectal examination as well. In many cases, he will arrange special abdominal X-rays—most commonly a barium enema, a barium meal or a cholecystogram (gall bladder X-ray). It's also now possible to look far in to either end of your alimentary tract with flexible telescope-like devices.

Commoner causes of chronic abdominal pain are dealt with under the following headings: ULCERS, GALL BLADDER (*see* A–Z of Parts of the Body), HIATUS HERNIA, and DIVERTICULAR DISEASE.

Acute Abdominal Pain

This is most commonly due to some trivial cause, such as indigestion or gastro-enteritis. Except in the occasional case of very hardy and stubborn individuals, it is rare for a person to ignore a serious cause of acute abdominal pain for long. Most of the important abdominal conditions pro-ducing acute pain will make their presence felt so forcibly that most patients will call the doctor in plenty of time. If in doubt, phone him and describe the symptoms. *Always* call the doctor if sudden pain causes collapse, or if severe pain persists for several hours.

UPPER ABDOMINAL PAIN. Acute and severe pain in the upper part of the abdomen may quite often be due to an ulcer, to gall bladder disease, or to inflammation of the pancreas.

LOIN AND FLANK PAIN. Acute pain in the loin, often running round to the groin, may be caused by kidney trouble (*see* KIDNEYS in the A–Z of Parts of the Body). The commonest such kidney condition is *acute pyelitis* (see PYELITIS); it is usually associated with a raised tempera-ture, shivering attacks, backache, and often frequent pass-ing of water. *Renal colic* is a severe griping pain produced by a stone which is formed in the kidney and which forces its way down the urinary tract.

CENTRAL ABDOMINAL PAIN. Acute and really severe pain in the central part of the abdomen may be due to a variety of causes. The commonest is probably appendicitis: this pain tends, after some hours, to shift into the lower right corner of the abdomen.

LOWER ABDOMINAL PAIN. Acute pain in the lower central part of the abdomen may be due to cystitis (*see* CYSTITIS).

Pain in the lower right hand side may, as we've seen above, be due to appendicitis. It may also be due to acute salpingitis (*see* SALPINGITIS), which is inflammation of the Fallopian tube. This condition may be suspected if there is fever, menstrual irregularity and vaginal discharge.

The other common cause of acute pain in the lower right side is a ruptured ectopic pregnancy (*see* ECTOPIC PREGNANCY). The chief symptoms of this condition are *(i)* missed periods; *(ii)* abdominal pain, followed within a few hours by *(iii)* vaginal bleeding.

Pain in the lower left side of the abdomen may also be due to either salpingitis or to an ectopic pregnancy, or to acute diverticulitis (*see* DIVERTICULAR DISEASE), which is characterized by fever and a prior history of bowel disturbances.

ABORTION
Illegal Abortion

Deliberate abortion was almost always carried out illegally until quite recent times. This meant that it became the province of the back-street operator—usually a cowboy (or cowgirl) with little or no knowledge of hygiene. There are still many such people around—not just in countries where abortion is still forbidden by law, but in areas where expense and other factors make it difficult for less well-off girls and women to obtain a legal termination of pregnancy.

I can't stress too strongly that no pregnant woman should ever consider going to one of these back-street operators, no matter how desperate her plight seems. *She may even be killed by the abortionist's efforts.* However, it's much more likely that she will suffer intense pain, heavy blood loss, and serious infection. Her health may be crippled, and she may become sterile. Although some women certainly do escape unscathed from the unqualified abortionist's hands, most run into trouble of some sort.

It goes almost without saying that attempts at self-abortion are just as dangerous. Women buy all sorts of preparations from the chemist and take them by mouth or place them in the vagina. These methods are unlikely to damage the baby, but they may seriously harm the mother.

Legal Abortion

THE LAW. Many countries have recently introduced laws to allow doctors to perform therapeutic termination of pregnancy. The situation varies greatly in different parts of the world; however, legal abortion is allowed in Great Britain but not in Northern Ireland or Eire.

In Britain, the law contains certain safeguards and provisos intended (*a*) to ensure that demands for termination are not made frivolously, and (*b*) to protect the expectant mother—there are, unfortunately, all too many thugs and shady characters who are ready to exploit a woman's distress for money.

PROCEDURE. If you think that you are pregnant, and you feel that your case merits a termination, you must act with considerable speed. When your period is 14 days overdue, have a urinary pregnancy test performed (preferably arranged by your doctor). Bear in mind that these tests are not 100% accurate—this is why it's best to have medical advice right from the start.

In any case, you will now have to consult a doctor who will assess whether you are eligible for termination. While it's desirable for you to see your own GP who may know your home background, you are not obliged to do so.

If in doubt, contact one of the charitable pregnancy services, like the British Pregnancy Advisory Service (their headquarters are at 58 Petty France, London SW1, tel: 01-222 0985), who will arrange a medical opinion. *Warning:* beware of 'advice services' whose purpose is to extract the maximum amount of money from you.

When the doctor you consult has examined you and discussed your reasons for wanting a termination, he will tell you whether he is willing to recommend one. If he is not willing, then you should consider whether it would be advisable to see another doctor instead.

Above all, don't delay. It is difficult to terminate pregnancies when more than 12–14 weeks have passed since the beginning of the last period—six weeks will already have elapsed by the time you are certain you are pregnant.

THE OPERATION. Once legally 'accepted' for a termination, you will be given a date on which to attend the hospital or approved clinic. If no more than about 12–14 weeks have elapsed, it will be relatively easy to terminate the pregnancy by the vaginal route. If the pregnancy has gone on for longer, however, a more extensive operation (often involving making an incision in the abdomen or inducing

a sort of 'mini-labour' by injections) will be necessary. Doctors are usually reluctant to perform terminations as late as this.

It's essential to realize that abortion by either of these methods is usually a procedure which requires full medical preparation. A woman, who's having an abortion during the early stages of pregnancy (before 14 weeks), should go into hospital or clinic the day before the operation and be carefully examined by a doctor to see that she is fit for a general anaesthetic. In the morning she will be prepared for the theatre and given a 'pre-med'. Once she has been anaesthetized, the surgeon will usually carry out the abortion by using a device called the Karman catheter to suck out the tiny blob of womb contents.

Afterwards, the patient is taken back to the ward, where she should normally remain for at least 24 hours.

However, a few clinics and hospitals—with Department of Health approval—do now allow selected patients home the same day.

ABRASIONS

Minor skin abrasions rarely give trouble if the skin is washed carefully with soap and warm water. Virtually any of the standard proprietary antiseptics can then be applied, followed (if the graze is extensive) by an adhesive dressing. *Warning*: any break in the skin can lead to infection with tetanus (lockjaw) unless immunization against this disease is up to date (*see* LOCKJAW).

ABSCESSES

These are collections of pus which occur in various parts of the body. In general, abscesses are treated according to the old surgical precept: "Where there is pus, let it out." Incision and drainage should, of course, be left to a doctor.

ACNE

This skin condition is extremely common, particularly among boys and girls in their teenage years. It is largely dependent on the balance of various hormones in the body, and, not surprisingly, usually settles down when adolescence is over. (Though not always, alas!)

The condition is associated with greasiness of the skin, which leads to blocking of the pores with oil. Germs become trapped in these blocked pores and as a result inflamed pustules develop on the face, shoulders, chest or back. In very severe cases, permanent scarring of the skin may result.

People with mild acne (and particularly teenagers) often try to treat the condition themselves with proprietary

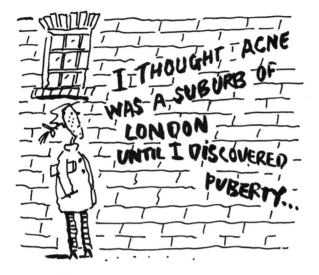

It seems likely that it works by stimulating the brain to produce certain natural pain-killers called 'endorphins'. Certainly, it can be highly effective in relieving pain, and a large number of NHS Pain Clinics are now using it for this purpose. Operations can also sometimes be carried out under acupuncture. Furthermore, there is some evidence that the technique can be used to relieve withdrawal symptoms in people who are addicted to heroin or nicotine.

Unfortunately, as yet there is no real evidence for the Chinese belief that acupuncture can be used to *cure* disease, as opposed to relieving symptoms.

ADDICTION (*See* DRUGS)

ALCOHOL—ABUSE OF

Alcohol, like nicotine, is, of course, one of the socially accepted drugs (*see* DRUGS). This does not, however, mean that it is harmless—far from it. Though most people learn to use and appreciate alcohol with reason and moderation, a percentage of the population do not. The results include widespread road deaths and injuries, wife-beating, unwanted pregnancy, drunkenness and the crimes that go with it, and chronic alcoholism. About half a million British people are thought to have an alcohol problem.

Acute Alcoholism

Acute alcoholism is simply the medical term for getting drunk. In most countries an occasional bout of such over-indulgence is socially acceptable, particularly among the young. There is no evidence that, within reason, this does any serious harm to the body (though an athlete in training should obviously avoid these excesses). Repeated or regular drunkenness, however, is *very* bad for the health.

In addition, there are certain dangers in acute intoxication with alcohol. Firstly, some people are unwise enough to take drink in combination with sleeping pills or certain other medicines: *this could be lethal*. Secondly, really prodigious drunkenness (*i.e.* to the point of unconsciousness) may quite often cause death, usually because of inhalation of vomit. Finally, there's the well-known risk to life and limb from road accidents. Even very small quantities of alcohol in the bloodstream will seriously impair road sense and co-ordination. It is very important to impress on the young that, quite apart from legal considerations, it is suicidal (or homicidal) to drink and drive—as any surgeon who has to patch up shattered bodies on a Saturday night (or certify them dead) can testify.

remedies. This is pointless. Acne should be treated by a doctor. A recent survey showed that most of these proprietary remedies are utterly worthless.

Therapy may have to be very prolonged, as there is no quick answer to acne. Some GPs refer severe cases to a dermatologist. Treatment usually includes prolonged use of tetracycline, often over a period of many months, exposure to sunlight or to ultra-violet light from a lamp, and the application of steroid and antibiotic skin preparations. Some dermatologists claim good results from putting female patients on the Pill. In the few severe cases with scarring and pitting, a process called 'dermabrasion', which is rather similar to 'sanding down', will often restore the skin to smoothness. A new product containing a vitamin A derivative is giving good results.

Good general measures are washing the face frequently with medicated soap, getting plenty of sunshine, and (at all costs) avoiding touching or picking the nose. The nose is a potent source of germs, and it may be necessary to use an antiseptic cream inside the nostrils. (*See also* PIMPLES.)

ACUPUNCTURE

The Chinese art of alleviating pain and treating disease by inserting needles at various points in the skin. Western doctors used to laugh at the whole idea of acupuncture, but on a recent trip to Hong Kong, during which I did a film report on the subject for BBC-TV, I was surprised to be shown convincing evidence that acupuncture does have a scientific basis.

Chronic Alcoholism

INCIDENCE. Chronic alcoholism is a form of addiction much like any other type of drug abuse (*see* DRUGS). In most Western countries, alcohol addiction is extremely common—far more so than misuse of either opiates (heroin and morphine) or LSD. It probably affects about five hundred thousand people in Britain. From that staggering figure, it should be obvious that the traditional belief that only depraved and morally corrupt people become alcoholic is absolute nonsense.

There is at present no way of forecasting whether a person is likely to become an alcoholic or not. Factors such as an unhappy childhood or serious personality difficulties are, of course, likely to increase the chance of alcoholism in later life. In many patients, however, there are other factors operating which we simply do not understand, and the fact remains that even respectable and apparently well-adjusted individuals can become alcoholics.

The long-term consequences of chronic alcoholism are disastrous. Work, family and social life are liable to be completely ruined. Serious mental disorder may well put the victim in a psychiatric hospital. Cirrhosis of the liver can occur after a period of years, and this may well prove fatal (*see* CIRRHOSIS). Some patients end up as vagrants and vagabonds; others simply drink themselves into an early grave.

TREATMENT. However, the alcoholic *can* be helped. Recognition of this fact by the patient and his relatives is of tremendous importance. In the old days, alcoholics were often virtually abandoned as so much human jetsam; medical treatment often consisted in simply telling them to pull themselves together.

Nowadays, this is not good enough. Help is available, and use should be made of it. Of prime importance is the fact that the patient must recognize that he is an alcoholic, and want to seek medical help. Many people refuse to make this admission until they have come near to ruining their lives. A wife who is worried about her husband's drinking habits should insist that he sees the family doctor who, if he feels that the patient is genuinely an alcoholic, will normally refer him for psychiatric help.

This isn't the place to discuss methods of psychiatric treatment, except to say that these methods are often successful in rehabilitating the patient. Also of great value is the work of the Alcoholics Anonymous organization, which has helped thousands of men and women to lead normal lives again.

Once off drink, the alcoholic should stay off it completely. Allowing even one glass of beer will probably start the patient off on a wild binge. I'm afraid that a good deal of back-sliding of this sort can be expected in most cases. However, where the alcoholic has the love and understanding of his family, coupled with proper psychiatric care and perhaps the support of the Alcoholics Anonymous organization, he stands a reasonable chance of complete rehabilitation and subsequently a happy and successful life. You can phone Alcoholics Anonymous between 10 a.m. and 10 p.m. every day at the London Region Telephone Service 01-834 8202. They will also put you in touch with a branch in your area. An alcoholic's family can get help through Al-Anon (01-403 0888).

ALLERGIES

An allergy is basically a state of unusual sensitivity to some foreign material—for instance, pollen, house dust, animal hairs, feathers, kapok (cushion stuffing), drugs, or certain foods.

In general, what happens in an allergic reaction is that the body is exposed to an agent called an 'antigen', and though this produces no obvious untoward effects at the time, substances called 'antibodies' are produced in response. On the next occasion that the body is exposed to the same antigen (whether it's grass pollen, animal hair or some type of food), the union of antigen and antibody is liable to produce dramatic effects—an urticarial skin rash, an asthma attack, or a bout of hay fever.

Many people experience skin or other allergies at some time in their lives. In a number of families, however, there is a marked hereditary tendency to several allergic diseases —notably eczema, hay fever, dust allergy and asthma. In such families, a child may have infantile eczema as a baby, and 'exchange' it for asthma as he grows older.

Fortunately, antihistamine drugs, desensitization techniques and other methods are nowadays available for the relief of allergies. (*See also* ASTHMA; ECZEMA; HAY FEVER; and URTICARIA.)

ALOPECIA

Alopecia literally means baldness, but, in practice, the word almost always indicates the conditions of ALOPECIA AREATA and ALOPECIA TOTALIS.

The former is very common in children; small patches of hair fall out of the scalp, often after an illness or an emotional upset. Dermatological treatment usually leads to regrowth of hair on the bald patch. It is important to distinguish the condition from ringworm, which sometimes gives a similar appearance.

Alopecia totalis is fortunately rare; it involves loss of all the hair on the head, including the eyebrows. The finger-nails may also be affected. Prolonged medical treatment may be necessary. Application of primula leaves has recently given some encouraging results.

AMNESIA

Amnesia is loss of memory. Contrary to what you see in the films, most cases are not due to a blow on the head, though it is true that severe head injuries do often produce a short period of 'retrograde amnesia'—that is, the victim cannot recall either being struck on the head, or the events which led up to the blow.

Amnesia in the sense of being unable to recall one's past

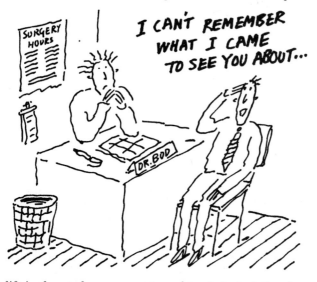

life is almost always a symptom of psychological disorder, and it is usual to find that the patient has adopted this defence mechanism to escape from problems with which he or she cannot cope. Such people are not malingerers and quite genuinely believe in their own symptoms. With help and understanding, they can usually be returned to health.

AMPHETAMINE, ABUSE

Amphetamines, or 'pep pills', were widely prescribed in the 1960s and 1970s as stimulants and alleged aids to slimming. Before long, they were being widely abused, mainly by middle-aged housewives, but latterly by young people as well. Unhappily, it took many years before really strict controls began to be imposed on the use of the drugs.

There are many types of amphetamine preparation still available. Colloquial names for these drugs include 'dexies',

'black bombers', 'black and tans', 'purple hearts', and 'French blues'.

I can't stress too firmly that all pep pills are very dangerous indeed, though individually they vary in risk.

Amphetamines taken by mouth increase energy and induce a feeling of well-being, which is why they are popular with tired housewives and teenage partygoers. Unfortunately, larger and larger doses of the pep pills are required to produce this effect.

While undoubtedly some people take these pills as a passing phase and then abandon them, others become 'hooked'. When someone reaches the stage of taking, say, 100 amphetamine pills a day and still requires more to get 'high', the temptation to change to heroin or morphia is obvious. Excessive use of amphetamines may also lead to psychosis (*i.e.* frank madness), and many people have been admitted to mental hospital suffering from this reaction.

In many ways, it is unfortunate that the immense amount of police and Customs time that has recently been directed to the control of cannabis (*see* CANNABIS) has not been applied instead to the stamping out of amphetamine abuse. (*See also* DRUGS.)

ANAEMIA

Anaemia is weakness of the blood. More strictly speaking, it is lack of the iron-containing blood pigment haemoglobin, which carries oxygen from the lungs to the various parts of the body.

There are literally dozens of different types of anaemia, some of the more important of which are dealt with under separate headings (*see* PERNICIOUS ANAEMIA; SICKLE CELL ANAEMIA; PREGNANCY). Far and away the commonest type, however, is simple iron-deficiency anaemia.

Iron Deficiency

CAUSES. This may be caused by lack of iron in the diet (particularly where people eat little meat). It is also seen in patients who have been losing iron through chronic blood loss, and is thus much commoner in women than in men. Women lose considerable quantities of iron in their periods, and may also do so if much bleeding occurs during the process of childbirth. In addition, the unborn baby extracts large quantities of iron from the mother for its own use.

Among men, the commonest cause of iron-deficiency anaemia is probably chronic blood loss due to ulcers (*see* ULCERS). Over-use of aspirin preparations (*see* ASPIRIN —ABUSE AND POISONING) and the presence of worms can cause chronic intestinal bleeding, too. Bleeding piles are also a possible cause of anaemia.

SYMPTOMS AND TREATMENT. The symptoms of ordinary iron-deficiency anaemia include paleness of the skin and of the red margin inside the lower eyelid, tiredness, breathlessness, giddiness, and occasionally angina (*see* ANGINA). The finger nails may become spoon-shaped.

Treatment is straightforward, once the diagnosis is made. A blood test will be required to exclude other causes of anaemia. Iron is given either by mouth or, in severe cases, by injection. Very gross anaemia will necessitate blood transfusion. The condition causing the anaemia must, of course, be corrected—for instance, a woman with very heavy periods may need hormone therapy or possibly a hysterectomy.

ANGINA
Angina is pain originating in the heart and brought on by exertion or excitement. Usually the pain starts in the central or upper part of the chest, and may spread down the left arm. Stopping the exertion should relieve the angina within a minute or two.

This symptom usually indicates degenerative change in the coronary arteries, which supply blood to the heart. Treatment varies in individual cases, but will usually include the use of trinitrin tablets which should be placed under the tongue just before commencing any exertion. They have a protective effect which lasts only for a matter of minutes.

But newer drugs have proved of considerable value in reducing the incidence of angina. The best known of these drugs are propranolol and oxprenolol.

Surgery is now offering new hope to a few angina sufferers. Already, it is sometimes possible to graft a length of vein (taken from elsewhere in the body) on to the heart to replace a damaged section of coronary artery, and also to widen a narrowed coronary artery with a 'balloon' inserted *via* an artery in the arm. (*See also* ARTERIES—HARDENING OF.)

ANKYLOSING SPONDYLITIS
Also known as 'poker back', this condition is quite common in men, but rare in women. It sometimes runs in families. Tall, slender men with a particular 'tissue type' (rather like a blood group) are most frequently affected. The early symptoms are low back pain and slight stiffness of the spine in the mornings. Eventually this stiffness becomes very marked so that the patient has difficulty in bending either forwards or sideways. Joints other than those of the spine may be affected, and a small proportion of patients develop eye, heart and other complications.

Treatment involves physiotherapy, the use of a hard, level bed at night and the administration of various pain-relieving and anti-inflammatory drugs. Ultrasonic treatment and radiotherapy to the spine are sometimes helpful.

APPENDICITIS
This is one of the most common of all surgical conditions, and in many countries about one in ten of the population bears an appendix scar.

It used to be generally accepted that there were various types of appendicitis—acute, subacute, recurrent and chronic. In recent years, however, doubt has been cast on the idea that the appendix can produce long-standing pain over a period of weeks, months or years. In practice all we need consider here is acute appendicitis.

Acute Appendicitis
SYMPTOMS. This pain is often generalized or centred round the navel to start with. Not long after it starts, the patient usually feels sick, and may well vomit once or twice (rarely more). He loses his appetite completely—a child or adult who still wants to tuck into his supper rarely has genuine appendicitis.

There is usually no diarrhoea, which helps to distinguish the condition from the vomiting and mild abdominal pain that characterize ordinary gastro-enteritis.

In fact, the bowels are usually slightly constipated. In years gone by, this used to mislead many parents into attempting treat their sick children with laxatives. Fortunately, people have more sense these days, and this dangerous practice is now much less common.

As the hours go by, the pain usually localizes in the lower right-hand corner of the abdomen. The wall of the belly becomes rigid and tender, and by now the patient feels really unwell. His temperature is slightly raised (to about 99.5°F or 37.5°C), his tongue is furred, and his breath often has a slightly unpleasant smell. At this stage, most people call the doctor.

TREATMENT. Once the diagnosis is made, the patient is usually operated on within a matter of hours. The inflamed appendix is removed and the abdomen stitched up, the whole process taking perhaps fifteen minutes. The patient will usually have to spend a week or so in hospital, and should take things easily for a couple of months afterwards.

ARTHRITIS (ARTHROSIS)
This word simply means 'joint inflammation'. Arthritis is therefore not a disease in itself.

Many patients become quite frightened by the word,

since they imagine that arthritis always means some kind of dread and crippling disorder. For this reason, doctors often prefer to use vague terms like 'rheumatism' and 'fibrositis' in preference to 'arthritis'.

There are many forms of arthritis, including ankylosing spondylitis (*see* ANKYLOSING SPONDYLITIS) and gout (*see* GOUT). There is also rheumatoid arthritis (*see* RHEUMATOID ARTHRITIS), and by far the most frequently encountered of all is osteoarthritis, or degenerative joint disease.

Osteoarthritis (DJD)

FEATURES. Osteoarthritis affects about half the population by the age of 60; approximately 98% of people aged 70 are said to have it to some degree. It's therefore almost a universal condition in the eldery. The patient with osteoarthritis needn't think that he is going to be crippled by it: in the majority of cases it is simply a matter of the joints 'not being as young as they used to be'. Admittedly, an unlucky minority of patients *do* become severely handicapped by arthritis.

TREATMENT. The joints that are principally affected by pain and swelling are those that bear the weight of the body—particularly the knees and the hips. The first principle of treatment, therefore, is to avoid being overweight.

Drugs are certainly of some value in osteoarthritis. Aspirin and the new 'anti-inflammatories' do reduce pain and inflammation, though they are not curative. Cortisone and the other steroid drugs are of no use in this condition (though they are in *rheumatoid arthritis*).

Physiotherapy is helpful. Affected joints should be given gentle exercise and massage, while heat treatment may also be of value. The patient should never allow the joints to become stiff through inactivity.

Surgical treatment of severe osteoarthritis is increasingly successful nowadays, though at present only a very small proportion of patients with the condition are operated on. These are mainly people with such gross arthritis of the hip or knee that they cannot walk: the results of the operation are superb, but the waiting lists are very long.

ASPIRIN—ABUSE AND POISONING

Abuse

Although aspirin is a useful drug, a substantial proportion of the population take excessive amounts of it. Let me make clear that we are not just talking about 'ordinary' aspirin tablets, but also about the many proprietary pain-killers which contain the drug.

Although the names of these preparations vary considerably, and though manufacturers sometimes seem to go to considerable lengths to conceal from the public the fact that the main ingredient of their product is simply cheap aspirin, it is always possible to detect this fact by looking at the side of the packet where the words 'Acid Acetylsalicyl.' or a similar abbreviation will be found.

Impressive claims such as 'containing the ingredients that 95% of doctors voted the most useful of all analgesics in medical history' invariably turn out to mean 'containing aspirin'.

It's also worth bearing in mind that certain standard medical preparations, such as ordinary codeine compound tablets, contain appreciable quantities of aspirin.

'Soluble' and 'junior' aspirins are just as open to abuse as the other types. The claim that 'doctors prefer' soluble aspirin is rather doubtful. Some do, some don't.

Prolonged use of all aspirin preparations is dangerous because of the effect the drug has on the lining of the stomach. It irritates this sensitive tissue, and may cause bleeding or ulcers. Many doctors believe that a high proportion of people admitted to hospital with vomiting of blood have been using excessive amounts of aspirin.

In general, the maximum dose for an adult should be two aspirins every six hours for two or three days, and this should not be exceeded without medical advice. The drug is best taken after meals.

Never take aspirin preparations for abdominal pain, and stop taking them if they give you indigestion. Anyone with a history of ulcer or chronic dyspepsia should avoid aspirin altogether. Alternative and reasonably safe preparations such as paracetamol are available.

Poisoning

Overdosage with aspirin is quite common, either in suicide attempts or where accidental poisoning has occurred in children: to avoid risk, keep bottles of aspirin under lock and key at all times. Remember the risk of children getting at 'junior' aspirin (see above).

TREATMENT. Although the patient often looks and feels well, death may be near. Aspirin poisoning is notoriously deceiving: however small the overdose or however well the patient feels, insist on immediate action. Firstly, make him vomit. Secondly, take him to hospital where, if he has digested any significant quantity of the drug, he will have a stomach wash-out and be admitted for observation.

ASTHMA

A chest disorder characterized by intermittent bouts of wheezing and breathlessness. These symptoms are due to transient narrowing of the air passages leading to the lungs, and to partial blockage of these passages by mucus or inflammatory swelling.

Asthma is basically an allergic condition (*see* ALLERGIES), but individual attacks may be triggered off not only by exposure to, say, dust or pollen, but by respiratory infections or psychological stress. The relative importance of the three factors (allergy, infection and mental stress) is uncertain, and in some patients stress may be of little or no importance.

Asthma, like other allergic conditions, tends to run in families. Often, one or other parent of an asthmatic child will have hay fever or eczema. The basic reasons why a person becomes asthmatic are not known, however.

Treatment

PREVENTIVE ACTION. The patient should be encouraged not to think of himself as an invalid. Asthmatic children should lead healthy, outdoor lives, with lots of sun, fresh air, and activity.

Coughs and respiratory infections should be treated promptly, however. Most asthmatics are given a short course of an antibiotic such as penicillin at the first sign of a bacterial throat or chest infection. Naturally, no asthmatic should ever smoke.

Substances to which the patient may be allergic (*e.g.* dust, feathers, pollen) should be avoided. They may be difficult to identify, however. Where no specific agent can be incriminated, the patient should avoid dusty atmospheres, and should try clearing his bedroom of feather quilts and pillows, horsehair mattresses, or unnecessary draperies. Sorbo rubber pillows and mattresses are unlikely to contain allergy-provoking substances.

Recent work in England and Holland shows that it is the presence of a tiny mite in housedust that provokes some asthma attacks.

Breathing exercises are of value in warding off bouts of asthma; they should be practised regularly each day.

TREATMENT BY DRUGS. Prevention of attacks by means of drugs may be attempted if the above general measures are not successful. ACTH injections and steroid tablets (such as prednisone) may be helpful. The steroids have very dangerous side-effects, however, so that their use must be very strictly supervized.

In recent years, new preparations have become available. Cromoglycate or Intal is taken from a special inhaler, usually four times a day, and seems to provide appreciable protection against asthmatic attacks. Some patients mistakenly try to use the drug as a treatment for acute attacks,

but this is not its purpose at all—it is purely a preventative.

Becotide is another invention of recent years: it's a steroid *inhaler* which is relatively free of the dangers of steroid tablets. Other similar steroid inhalers are now on the market, as are some promising new oral anti-asthma tablets.

ATHLETE'S FOOT

This is a fungus infection of the skin, which spreads rapidly among people who go barefoot on moist floors. It is thus often picked up in games changing-rooms, dormitories, showers, etc.

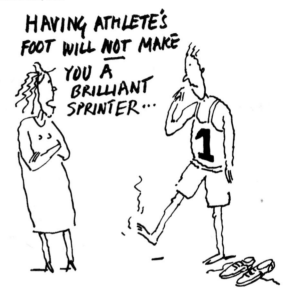

The fungus, for some unknown reason, almost invariably attacks the gaps on either side of the fourth toe, though it may spread to other toes, and often to the crutch area.

Treatment used to be tedious and unsatisfactory, but is nowadays very straightforward, since agents like chlorphenesin ointment will clear up the condition entirely in a few days. Admittedly, it does tend to recur...and recur... and recur.

AUTISM

This is a form of mental disorder which occurs in early childhood. It is said to affect 4 in every 10,000 children. Some authorities describe it as an infantile form of schizophrenia, but many others dispute this view.

As a rule, the child appears normal up until well into the first year of life. His parents may then notice that he shows no signs of interest or pleasure on being picked up or cuddled.

As a toddler, the child makes no real attempt to talk or to interest himself in adults or other children. He seems, quite literally, to be living in a mental world of his own. Despite this extreme coldness to the human environment, the autistic child may be aggressive and hostile when crossed. He may have set rituals which he likes to perform each day, and if these are interfered with he may become quite uncontrollable.

These symptoms are, of course, immensely distressing for the parents of autistic children, but many of them find that with love and understanding, they can manage to 'get through' to their children in some degree.

There is, however, no real cure for autism. Some autistic children can nevertheless be greatly helped by special education with a maximum of individual supervision. Speech therapy will be particularly helpful. In some countries parents of autistic children have formed national associations and established special residential schools for sufferers from this disorder.

B

BACKACHE

This is one of the commonest of all symptoms encountered in medical practice. Precise diagnosis is often difficult, since the back is such a complex region of the body, with dozens of bones, muscles and ligaments in close proximity to each other.

Fortunately, most conditions causing backache are relatively short-lived, and get better after a reasonable period of rest. Where pain persists, there must, of course, be full investigation, including X-rays of the spine.

The commonest causes of backache are thought to be minor muscle and ligament strains. Also sometimes encountered is osteoarthritis of the spine (DJD). This tends to wax and wane, perhaps giving trouble once or twice a year for a period of a few days. This type of arthritis is discussed further under the heading ARTHRITIS.

Persistent low backache and morning stiffness in a young man suggest ankylosing spondylitis or 'poker back' (see ANKYLOSING SPONDYLITIS).

In a young woman, low backache is more likely to be caused by lifting heavy weights: this symptom is common in nurses.

Backache in women is all too frequently ascribed to womb disorders or other gynaecological troubles. However, a woman with backache usually has something wrong with her back, and not her reproductive organs.

'Slipped Disc'

'Slipped disc' is a fairly common cause of backache. In reality, a disc doesn't 'slip'. What actually happens is that discs (which are cartilaginous shock-absorbers forming cushions between the bones of the spine) are liable to protrude backwards and press on nerve roots.

This protrusion often happens when the patient is bending over, or lifting a heavy weight. In 80% of cases, it occurs in the small of the back, though protrusions also occur in the neck region.

Characteristically, the victim feels a sudden and quite severe pain, and may have difficulty in standing up straight. Later, the pain usually runs down the back of one or other leg as far as the foot. (This symptom is known as SCIATICA.)

Treatment initially consists of confinement to bed until the symptoms improve. A hard, flat mattress should be used. A plaster jacket may sometimes have to be worn for several months. Under certain circumstances, operation on the spine may be necessary to remove the prolapsed disc.

Manipulation—by a doctor, a physiotherapist or an osteopath—often helps. So too may an epidural injection of local anaesthetic—that is, an injection into the base of the spine. Traction of the spine can also be helpful.

BAD BREATH

Bad breath, or halitosis, is a relatively common condition. Fortunately, in most people it is only an occasional and passing problem.

Far and away the most frequently encountered causes of bad breath are cigarette smoking and dental decay. The remedy for the first is to give up smoking, and the remedy for the second is to clean the teeth regularly and to see a dentist. Antiseptic mouthwashes have some marginal benefit, and, like toothpaste, are often pleasantly scented.

Digestive upsets are not now thought to be a common cause of bad breath, though certain acute abdominal conditions (see APPENDICITIS) will produce a type of halitosis for a few hours. Eating highly-flavoured foods, such as curry and garlic, is much more likely to produce an offensive pong! A similar phenomenon is often noticeable during a hangover, of course.

Finally, one or two chronic lung diseases (*see* BRON-CHIECTASIS) produce a very unpleasant aroma on the breath, because of pus in the air passages.

BALDNESS

Baldness of varying degrees is extremely common among the male population. Ordinary male frontal baldness is characterized by hair loss above the temples and on top of the scalp. It is a hereditary condition, being passed from father to son. If a man's father went bald early, it is quite likely that he will do so too.

What can be done about this? The answer, regrettably, is very little. And because of the concern it causes the balding man, it is not surprising that for centuries charlatans have grown fat on men willing to pay for 'scientific' methods of hair restoring. There is, apparently, no limit to the credulity of the man who is going bald and who is desperate to have something done about it. Hair tonics, hair restorers, hair lotions, scalp massage, scalp friction, electrical treatment —all are available, at a price, but all to no effect.

Treatment

Apart from buying a toupée, what can be done about male frontal baldness?

At present, there appear to be two possible answers—hair weaving and hair transplants.

Hair weaving is a process in which strands of human hair are attached to the remaining shafts on the scalp of

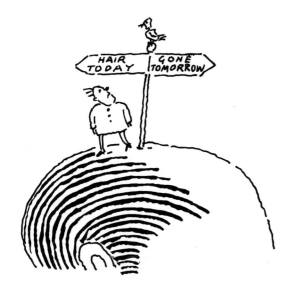

the bald person. The attachment is at skin level, and a skilful operator can produce a remarkably realistic impression of increased hair growth. Obviously, the subject has to have at least some hairs on the area which is to be treated, in order to provide attachment for the new ones. One drawback with hair weaving is that, as one's own hairs grow, the woven-in 'thatch' is slowly lifted off the scalp. Adjustments, therefore, have to be made every few months.

Anyone thinking of undergoing hair weaving should ask to see living proof of the efficiency of the operators at the clinic of his choice. (Photos of treated patients, can, of course, be very misleading.) In a business where big money is to be made, operating standards may vary considerably.

This remark applies with even more force to hair transplantation. There are a number of ways of carrying out this process—some more efficient, more expensive or more painful than others. In general, the plan is to remove hair from the neck or the back of the skull, and reimplant it on the bald patch. As techniques of hair transplantation become more efficient, this will certainly develop into the method of the future. But it's very, very expensive.

Nonetheless it is possible that hormone therapy may one day be utilized to prevent baldness. It should be emphasized that baldness does not, however, result from deficiency of male hormones, or lack of 'virility'. Indeed, there are some people who hold the contrary to be true, a thought which may be of some solace to the balding male!

Baldness occurring in women and children, or very sharply localized hair loss occurring in men, is usually due to some specific cause (such as emotional shock, or a fungus infection) and may respond well to treatment. (*See* ALOPECIA.)

BARBER'S ITCH

This is an inflammation of the beard area of the face. Red lumps and pus-filled 'spots' develop on the cheeks, chin and front of the neck. Shaving tends to make the condition worse since the razor clips the tops off the irregularities in the skin. Treatment should be undertaken by a doctor, and home remedies should not be applied to the skin. It may be necessary to stop shaving for a short period of time. If, as often happens, the condition is complicated by ringworm, an anti-fungal ointment will help. (*See* RINGWORM.)

BARBITURATES—ABUSE AND POISONING
Barbiturate Abuse

Barbiturates are a group of drugs used either as sedatives or as 'sleeping pills'. Common members of the group include phenobarbitone, Amytal, Soneryl, Nembutal and Seconal.

Though these drugs are very valuable, their abuse has

now become widespread. In the 1950s and 1960s, the dangers of dependence on barbiturates weren't obvious, and doctors accordingly prescribed them widely, both for people who could not sleep and (perhaps more important) for people who needed mild daytime sedation. Many of these patients have become more or less 'hooked', or dependent, on barbiturates. For some of them the dependence is not very serious and is easily broken, but others simply cannot get through a day without taking the drug.

Over the last few years, a nationwide anti-barbiturate campaign run by doctors has begun to take effect so that addiction to 'barbs' is becoming less common.

When the user reaches the stage of taking large doses, he is likely to spend much of his time in a slightly dazed condition. His speech and thoughts are slow, his judgement is poor, and he may tend to stumble a lot. Irritability and suicidal tendencies may follow. Accidental poisoning (see below) is very common at this stage, particularly if the patient takes any alcohol on top of his barbiturates. Withdrawal symptoms may be very serious, and even fatal.

Some teenagers have taken to barbiturates for 'kicks', though the appeal of the drugs is somewhat hard to understand, since they provide very little, if any, pleasure for the average person. Kids nickname these preparations 'barbs', 'goof-balls', or 'sleepers'. 'Purple hearts' and 'French blues' are barbiturate/amphetamine mixtures (*see* AMPHETAMINES—ABUSE OF).

A particular danger is that a few people have taken up the incredibly foolhardy practice of injecting crushed up pills or capsules into themselves. *This is sheer lunacy, and a short cut to death.*

TREATMENT. Obviously, it is best not to get 'hooked' on barbiturates in the first place. Anyone who thinks dependence is occurring in themselves or in one of the family should talk at once to their general practitioner. He will try to wean the patient off the drugs and, if this fails, will recommend specialist therapy.

Barbiturate Poisoning

This is common. Some cases are accidental but most are suicidal. About one in eight of all those admitted to hospital with barbiturate overdosage die, and others suffer irreparable brain damage. On the brighter side, many of those who recover never try to kill themselves again and, after proper psychiatric help, lead happy and useful lives. In other words, the widespread belief that there is little point in saving people who try to poison themselves 'as they'll only try to do it again' is complete nonsense.

TREATMENT. If the patient is conscious, make him vomit and then get him to hospital as rapidly as possible. If he is unconscious, call an ambulance. Delay in seeking medical aid greatly increases the risk of death.

BAT EARS

To have unusually prominent ears can be a very trying affliction for a child. The condition is congenital, and often runs in the family. It is *not* caused by sleeping on the ears as a baby.

In severe cases, a minor plastic operation should be considered. Taping the ears back at night is not helpful. If all else fails, think of Prince Charles or Clark Gable!

BEDSORES

These are liable to occur in anyone who is confined to bed for a long period of time—particularly if they are old and debilitated. A person who is able to move around in bed and who has good nursing care stands the best chance of avoiding bedsores. Patients who are unconscious or completely immobile are always at risk.

Therefore, anyone who is confined to bed should normally be encouraged to move his arms and legs around, and to lie on his side and on his stomach as well as on his back. Unconscious patients should lie on their sides, and be turned every hour. The pressure points of the body (the heels, the buttocks, the small of the back, the shoulder blades and the elbows) should be washed, dried and powdered twice a day. The doctor should be informed if any of these areas become reddened or sore, as ulceration is then likely to occur.

BED-WETTING

Bed-wetting (*nocturnal enuresis*) is a common condition. It is essential to realize that this disorder is obviously not the child's fault, since he is fast asleep at the time. It is therefore sheer folly to become annoyed with him or to punish him. Fortunately, it is now increasingly rare that one comes across the sort of mother who actually *beats* her child for wetting the bed, but many parents still insist on treating the child as though he had done something shameful.

When a child, who has been 'dry' for a considerable period of time, suddenly starts wetting the bed the cause is almost invariably emotional, and some kind of subconscious fear is usually found to be disturbing sleep. Resentment over a new baby and fears of loss of parental affection are probably the commonest sources of such upset.

In these circumstances, the parents should try to seek

out the cause of the unhappiness and do what they can to alleviate it. This is sometimes surprisingly easy: undemanding encouragement and the repeated gentle assurance that Mummy and Daddy still love the child can work wonders. If simple measures fail, however, consult a doctor.

In the case of a child who has simply never become 'dry' at all, the cause may again be psychological. A high proportion of such children do, however, have either a urinary infection or a structural abnormality of the urinary tract. Special laboratory tests and X-rays will be needed to discover these conditions.

But 'ordinary' cases of bed-wetting respond very well to the use of a special *bed-wetter alarm* which wakes the child the moment he starts to pass water. Your local Child Health Clinic may possibly have one available for loan. If not, you can buy one. Also new research has shown that hypnosis can help. *But there's no point in trying to 'treat' bed-wetting below the age of five, since up to this age it's statistically normal.*

BEE STINGS (*See* STINGS)

BELL'S PALSY

This is a sudden paralysis of the facial nerve, as a result of which the face becomes sharply drawn to one side. The cause of the condition is unknown. It is sometimes mistaken for a stroke.

No effective treatment was available until quite recent years. Nowadays, injections of ACTH (*corticotrophin*) are given daily for about two weeks. It is important that this treatment should be started within hours of the diagnosis being made. Recent reports suggest that steroid drugs by mouth may also be helpful.

BIRTHMARKS

Some form of minor birthmark is present on the skin of nearly all babies, though fortunately most of these marks are inconspicuous. Others seem very ugly at birth but will often shrink and become far less obvious as time goes by.

'Stork marks' are seen between the eyebrows and on the nape of the neck: they disappear in the first year of life.

Moles may be more disfiguring, particularly in a girl, but most of them can, if necessary, be removed by a surgeon when the child is older.

Port wine stains are very conspicuous, but smaller and lighter-coloured ones often fade as the years go by. Surgery is occasionally possible for larger port wine stains. The use of cosmetic preparations such as Covermark in teenage and adult life gives remarkable results. Occasionally, lasers

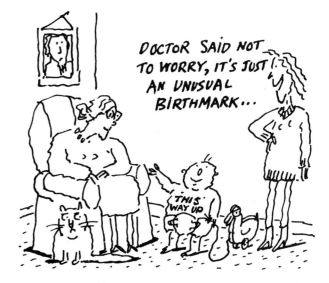

can be used to get rid of port wine stains.

Cavernous Haemangiomas ('strawberries') are basically collections of blood in the skin. They shrink and disappear during early childhood.

BLACKHEADS

These are collections of oily material in the pores of the skin. They can be pressed out with a special instrument (called a comedone extractor) which can be bought quite cheaply at a chemist. The fingers should not be used to squeeze blackheads as they can cause infection.

If a boy or a girl has a lot of blackheads, they've probably got acne, and they should be treated by a doctor (*see* ACNE).

BLOOD PRESSURE

People often say that they have 'blood pressure'. This doesn't mean a lot, since we all have a blood pressure, be it high, low, or normal.

In practice, low blood pressure is rare, except after a heart attack, or 'coronary'. However, lowered blood pressure does occur when people faint.

High blood pressure (hypertension) is very, very common indeed. There are various rather rare causes of hypertension, but the vast majority of cases are either 'essential' (meaning that we do not know the cause), or, less frequently, secondary to kidney disease. Kidney disease is sometimes curable, so that any youngish person who develops high blood pressure should have a full investigation of his kidney function, including X-rays (see KIDNEYS in the A–Z of Parts of the Body). Essential hypertension, on the other hand, tends to progress slowly, usually over a period of many years, and at present it cannot be cured.

Preventive treatment is very important, however, since it keeps the blood pressure down, reduces the incidence of complications, such as strokes, and greatly increases the life span. Treatment in each individual case must be determined by the patient's doctor, but the following points are of considerable value.

1. Keep the weight down. An overweight hypertensive patient who slims down to below average weight often finds that the blood pressure returns to near normal.
2. Keep salt intake down. Avoiding taking salt at the table is usually sufficient; there is rarely any point in dispensing with salt in cooking.
3. Maintain reasonable physical activity: the fitter a patient can keep by regular exercise (e.g. walking), the better.
4. Avoid smoking. Cigarettes increase the risk of coronary disease, a frequent complication of high blood pressure.
5. If urinary troubles occur, get prompt and thorough treatment (see CYSTITIS; URINARY DISORDERS).
6. Take the prescribed drug therapy every day. A very wide range of antihypertensive drugs are now available, and their use has greatly improved the outlook in this condition.
7. Think carefully before either becoming pregnant or going on the Pill—both can push the blood pressure up.

BOILS

It is usually best not to treat them yourself unless, for any reason, medical advice is not available. If this is the case, proceed as follows.

Where there is no 'head', simply place an adhesive dressing over the boil. Where there *is* a head, it may be pricked with a pin which has been sterilized in the flame of a match. The pus may then be gently pressed out. Do *not* squeeze a boil on the face, however. Wash the hands very carefully before and afterwards, and throw the contaminated pin and all cotton wool or other soiled dressings away. Cover the area with gauze or a sticking plaster.

N.B. No one with a boil should under any circumstances be allowed to prepare food (see FOOD POISONING.)

Recurrent boils raise the suspicion of diabetes. Take a specimen of urine to your doctor, who will test it for sugar.

BRONCHIECTASIS

This is a chronic respiratory condition which is caused by damage to the air passages leading to the LUNGS (see A–Z of Parts of the Body). Such damage commonly occurs as a complication of PNEUMONIA, WHOOPING COUGH, or MEASLES.

Typically, bronchiectasis starts in childhood. The boy or girl never really seems to make a good recovery from one or another of the diseases mentioned above, and thereafter is plagued by recurrent coughs which usually keep him or her off school for several months each year.

What has happened is that the damaged air passages have become grossly widened, providing a ready nesting place for germs. Pus collects in these passages and is coughed up in large quantities each morning.

Treatment is a complex business, involving physiotherapy, the use of antibiotics, and sometimes lung surgery. Postural drainage of the affected area of lung to drain out all the pus is of great importance.

BRONCHIOLITIS

This means inflammation of the smallest air passages leading to the LUNGS (see A–Z of Parts of the Body). The condition is very common in infants, and is caused by a virus infection. The disorder is more or less the equivalent of acute bronchitis (see BRONCHITIS) in adults or older children, and, like acute bronchitis, is usually followed by complete recovery.

BRONCHITIS

Bronchitis means inflammation of the large air passages leading to the lungs. The term is, however, used to describe two entirely different conditions—acute bronchitis and chronic bronchitis. Failure to realize this often leads mothers to become quite unnecessarily alarmed when told that their children have acute bronchitis—which is usually a fairly trivial condition, followed by complete recovery.

Acute Bronchitis

This may occur as a complication of colds, flu and other virus infections. There is tightness of the chest associated with a dry, painful cough. Later, a good deal of yellow sputum may be coughed up.

The patient should be in a moist atmosphere: the use of an old-fashioned steam kettle will help, but failing this, inhalations of steam from a basin will prove of value. Depending on the circumstances, the doctor may or may not prescribe antibiotics. In the great majority of cases, the patient is better within a few days.

Chronic Bronchitis

This entirely different disease is a long-standing inflammation of the respiratory tubes. Its main cause is cigarette smoking, though other factors are recurrent virus infections, air pollution, and obesity (*see* FATNESS).

Typically, the patient began smoking as a young man or woman, had a 'smoker's cough' fairly soon, and by the age of 40 was experiencing a moderately severe cough every winter. By the age of 50, he is likely to be rapidly heading downhill, with marked breathlessness, and persistent cough. In many cases, he becomes too disabled to work.

TREATMENT. There is no actual cure, but the disease can be arrested by

(i)   giving up smoking entirely;
(ii) avoiding smoky atmospheres;
(iii) obtaining prompt medical treatment at the slightest sign of a cold;
(iv) keeping the weight down;
(vi) in selected cases, using breathing exercises; and
(vi) regularly taking medicines prescribed by the doctor.

It cannot be stressed too strongly, however, that it is virtually pointless for a patient to take vast quantities of drugs if he persists in continuing to smoke. In this condition, every cigarette really is a nail in the coffin.

BRUCELLOSIS

Also known as undulant fever, this condition is usually caused by drinking milk infected with the germ Brucella. However, many veterinary surgeons, farm hands and slaughter-house workers are liable to infection simply through contact with cows. For the average person, the greatest danger is drinking unpasteurized milk—*i.e.* milk straight from the cow. The features of the disease are prolonged fever, headache, sweating and general ill-health.

BRUISES

Most bruises are better left alone without any treatment. There is not the slightest evidence that applying steaks to facial bruises does any good whatsoever. However, any cold compress will be useful in relieving pain—and the new 'cold packs' available at chemists are very helpful.

Extensive or painful bruising should be treated by a doctor, who will ensure that no more injury is present. He may give an enzyme preparation, such as Chymoral, to hasten absorption of the bruise.

BUNION

This is a swelling at the base of the big toe, caused by wearing tight shoes. Heat, rest and antibiotics are useful if a bunion becomes inflamed, but cure is only possible by means of surgery.

CANCER

This is the general term applied to any malignant growth. There is no single disease called cancer, since malignancy may occur in virtually any organ or tissue of the body. It's important to realize this fact, since people sometimes imagine that, because they have had a negative test for one type of cancer, they are safe from all the hundreds of other types. For instance, a woman who has had a negative 'Pap' smear (for cancer of the cervix, or neck of the womb) often assumes that this means she cannot have cancer of the breast. This is quite wrong.

What Happens

Cancer is essentially a process in which a cell 'goes mad', reproducing itself again and again until literally millions of cells have been formed from the original one, giving a mass of malignant tissue. This tissue usually has the characteristics of *(i)* invasiveness—it will eat its way through adjacent organs, and *(ii)* capacity for being spread to other parts of the body, usually via the bloodstream.

The causes of cancer are not fully understood. In some types of malignancy, however, it is clear that certain factors have played a very important part. The link between smoking and lung cancer is now well known, while certain forms of chronic inflammation may lead to cancer. A rare type of malignancy, seen almost only in Africa, is believed to be transmitted from man to man, possibly by viruses. Apart from this, however, cancer is never infectious.

Treatment

Treatment of cancer has improved out of all recognition in recent years. Unhappily, many people still believe, quite wrongly, that the diagnosis of cancer is a death warrant.

In fact, a very high proportion of patients whose cancer was diagnosed early now survive to lead happy and healthy lives. The operative word is 'early'. Again, because of our unfortunate failure to educate the public, the average cancer patient delays for several months after noticing symptoms before he seeks medical advice.

Possible Symptoms

Listed below, therefore, are the commonest symptoms of the most frequently encountered types of cancer. All adults should read the list and bear the symptoms in mind:

BOWEL: rectal bleeding; black motions; a sudden change in bowel habit; sometimes chronic abdominal pain.

BREAST: a lump in the breast.

CERVIX (neck of womb): bleeding after intercourse or between periods.

GULLET (oesophagus): inability to swallow food.

LARYNX: persistent unexplained hoarseness.

PROSTATE GLAND: inability to pass urine properly.

SKIN: unexplained ulcers: moles (particularly black moles) which are increasing in size or bleeding.

STOMACH: persistent upper abdominal pain; unexplained weight loss.

WOMB (body of): bleeding after the menopause; bloodstained or brown discharge before or after menopause.

I must stress that most of these symptoms may well indicate some quite benign condition. For instance, the symptoms of ordinary enlargement of the prostate gland and of cancer of the prostate are virtually identical: only special tests can distinguish between them (*see* PROSTATE in the A–Z of Parts of the Body). In addition, it is unfortunately true that many patients have one or other of the cancers mentioned above without symptoms. (This is why routine investigations such as 'Pap' smears are so valuable.)

These facts do not, however, invalidate the general principle: if you have any of the symptoms listed above, go and see your doctor as soon as possible. He will examine you, and tell you if further investigation is necessary. (Women are particularly advised to read the sections BREAST and CERVIX in the A–Z of Parts of the Body.)

CANNABIS (POT) USAGE

Still remarkably little is known about cannabis. This may surprise readers who have heard either (a) the fantastic and violent abuse heaped on the drug by opponents of it, or (b) the lyrical rhapsodizing of those who regard it as some sort of passport to instant happiness.

In fact, we know so little about its action that we still can't really say whether it is harmful. There is no convincing evidence either way at present, probably because there are dozens of different kinds of cannabis of varying strengths and purity, and so little research has been done that no satisfactory classification of the various types exists.

It is clear, however, that cannabis is not an addictive drug. This knowledge has only become widespread among doctors in the last few years, and even today many people do not realize the fact; some sections of the Press still continue to confuse cannabis with the highly dangerous and addictive drug heroin. In fact, heroin has no more in common with cannabis than it has with aspirin.

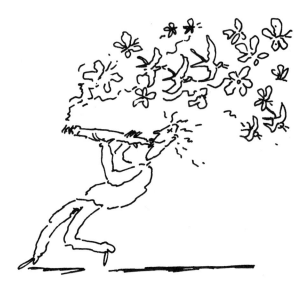

Pot smoking is of course very common among younger people. Parents who discover that their children have indulged in the practice shouldn't become in the least alarmed. They should, however, try to dissuade them from smoking pot again, for two very good reasons.

The first is that, as stated above, we don't know if the drug is harmful—there is certainly a small possibility that its use might lead some young people on to experimenting with such appallingly dangerous drugs as heroin.

The second reason is simple. In most Western countries, the legal penalties for possessing or passing on cannabis are at best severe, and at worse barbarous. Until such time, therefore, as we know more about the drug (and until such time as the law takes a rather more enlightened view of its use), it's best to be a bit wary about it.

CARBUNCLE

This is an acute inflammation of the tissues under the skin, caused by infection with the same germ that is found in boils. The commonest site is the nape of the neck. The treatment used to be surgical excision, but this is rarely necessary in these days of antibiotics.

CARTILAGE INJURIES

This type of knee injury is very common indeed, particularly among young men. Characteristically, the patient has been playing football or putting some other form of strain on the leg. Suddenly, he experiences intense pain in the knee. The leg may 'lock', so that he is unable to straighten it for some hours. The joint may become grossly swollen, but go down over a period of several days. The patient often thinks he is better but the knee 'goes' under him again sooner or later, with renewed pain, locking and swelling.

All these symptoms are caused by tearing of one or other of the two little pieces of cartilage (or gristle) that are found in the knee joint. Once torn, a cartilage cannot heal. The only treatment, therefore, is operation (usually to remove the torn cartilage). In a new and very effective procedure, torn bits of cartilage are removed with a telescope-like instrument. The earlier this is done the better, since it reduces the chances of osteoarthritis in later life. After the operation, the patient must work very hard at exercises to build up the leg muscles. The results of treatment are usually very good.

CATARACTS

A cataract is when the lens of the eye becomes opaque. Cataracts obstruct the light, which leads to failing vision or even sometimes blindness.

Where cataract is severe, the only treatment is surgical operation. Cataract operations were first performed in India about 1,000 BC. The modern operation involves removing the whole lens of the eye. Naturally, this means that glasses with powerful lenses have to be used instead. An alternative is to 'implant' lenses into the eye—or to use contact lenses. Vision may be distorted for some weeks after the operation, but most people achieve quite reasonable eyesight within a few months.

CATARRH

Persistent catarrh may be due to hay fever (*see* HAY FEVER) or related allergic conditions of the nose, to nasal malformations, and, in children, to enlargement of the adenoids. Most cases respond well to medical or surgical treatment.

CEREBRAL PALSY (*See* SPASTIC DISORDERS.)

CHANGE OF LIFE (*See* MENOPAUSE.)

CHEST DISORDERS (*See* ASTHMA, BRONCHIECTASIS, BRONCHIOLITIS, BRONCHITIS, COUGH, EMPHYSEMA, PLEURISY, PNEUMOCONIOSIS, PNEUMONIA, PULMONARY EMBOLISM, and TUBERCULOSIS.)

CHEST PAIN

Pain in the chest is a common symptom, but one which is often difficult to diagnose accurately.

Acute Chest Pain

In a person over the age of about 35 (and especially in a male), sudden severe central chest pain may be due to a 'coronary'. (*See* CORONARY THROMBOSIS.) The pain is crushing in nature and may run from the centre of the chest down the left arm. The sufferer is often sweating and shocked.

FIRST AID TREATMENT. Lie the patient down flat and keep him still but comfortable. Call a doctor or an ambulance. If breathing stops, give the 'kiss of life'; if the pulse or heartbeat cannot be felt, carry out cardiac massage. (*See* FIRST AID TECHNIQUES OF RESUSCITATION in the A–Z of Emergencies.)

OTHER CAUSES OF ACUTE CHEST PAIN. Most such pains, especially in young people, are due to trivial causes, *e.g.* indigestion or muscular strain. Pain below the left nipple is extremely common in young adults who are worried about their hearts; it is rarely of any significance at all, but check with your doctor.

Pain made worse by taking a deep breath may be due to pleurisy (*see* PLEURISY). Chest pain occurring in anyone who has been in bed for a few days may be due to pulmonary embolism (*see* PULMONARY EMBOLISM). In either case, medical help is needed.

Chronic Chest Pain

Long-standing pain in the chest may be due to a variety of conditions, some, though not all, of which are very serious. Full investigation, including a chest X-ray, is absolutely essential. Do not delay in consulting the doctor.

CHICKEN POX

This is a benign virus disease occurring mainly in children. The virus is probably identical with the one which causes shingles.

The incubation period is usually between 12 and 21 days. In most cases an itchy rash is the first sign that anything is wrong, though some children have headache and slight fever shortly before the spots appear.

The rash is thickest on the body, and sparsest at the hands and feet. It is first seen in the form of tiny red spots; these become filled with clear fluid, but the fluid soon turns to pus. Eventually, each spot dries up into a crust.

Complications of chicken pox are rare. There is no specific treatment for the condition. Most children are fit for school two weeks after the first appearance of the rash. Calamine helps relieve the dreaded itch!

CHILLS (*see* COLDS)

CHOLECYSTITIS (*See* GALL BLADDER, under A–Z of Parts of the Body.)

CHOLERA
Cholera is an acute infectious disease, characterized by very severe diarrhoea. The resultant loss of fluid may be fatal.

The condition is caused by a germ which is passed in the stools and transmitted via impure drinking water. In most of the underdeveloped and developing countries of the world human excreta contaminate the drinking water supplies to a greater or lesser extent. A similar situation existed in developed countries until late Victorian times, when stringent measures, taken to ensure the purity of drinking water, put a stop to cholera.

In the eastern part of the Indian sub-continent cholera has remained endemic for centuries, and 'waves' of it periodically spread out across much of the world. A particular strain of cholera (the 'El Tor' type) has advanced westwards in somewhat alarming fashion in the last decade. Some tourists from temperate countries have returned home from Spain and North Africa with the disease.

Fortunately, the state of the water and sanitation facilities in developed countries renders actual transmission of cholera fairly unlikely, though there may be danger where a food handler is involved.

Any person going to a 'cholera' country should obtain immunization from his doctor well beforehand. Bear in mind that cholera 'shots' only give partial protection and for a very limited time. Therefore, great care is necessary in avoiding contaminated food or water. Anyone who returns home suffering from severe diarrhoea after a trip to the East, or to Spain or North Africa, should have a laboratory test for cholera carried out immediately.

CHOREA (*See* ST VITUS' DANCE.)

CIRRHOSIS
This is a form of degeneration of the liver. There are many possible causes, but in adults the commonest form of cirrhosis is due to alcoholism. Persistent over-indulgence in alcohol, and especially wines and spirits, is responsible for the damage to the liver cells, though poor nutrition may play a part in the development of the condition. It is important to realize that one can become an alcoholic cirrhotic without ever actually getting drunk.

The main symptoms are general ill-health, loss of appetite,

nausea in the mornings, jaundice, and swelling of the abdomen and ankles. The patient usually admits that he tends to start drinking well before lunch and carry on through the day.

There is no actual cure for alcoholic cirrhosis, but, provided the patient is willing to give up drink, life can be greatly prolonged by the use of drugs and a suitable diet. If the victim doesn't stop drinking, episodes of coma, bleeding or mental confusion may necessitate urgent admission to hospital. (*See also* ALCOHOL—ABUSE OF.)

CLEFT PALATE
This is a common malformation, but fortunately one that can be readily helped by surgery. Some babies have a very mild degree of cleft palate, involving only the uvula (the little globe of tissue at the back of the throat) and the back part of the soft palate. In others, the gap extends forward into the hard palate so that there is open communication between the mouth and the nose. There may well be an associated hare lip (*see* HARE LIP). The baby will probably have some difficulty sucking in the early weeks of life, but with care it should be possible to feed him quite adequately. Surgery is usually postponed until a later stage of infancy when the parts of the palate are larger and easier to operate on.

COELIAC DISEASE
A childhood condition in which there is recurrent illness and failure to thrive. Characteristically, the child passes large, pale motions. Wasting may be very severe, and in years gone by the outlook of such children was appalling, many of them dying before adulthood.

Some years ago, however, research in Holland and the UK demonstrated that the disease was due to an abnormal sensitivity to gluten, the protein found in wheat, rye and barley. This defect is present in about one in 2,000 of the population, including some adults with the condition known as sprue.

The outlook has been revolutionized by this discovery. Affected children will grow strong and healthy, provided they keep to a gluten-free diet. Bakeries can provide parents with special bread, biscuits and flour. Further advice can be obtained from the national societies (like the Coeliac Society, PO Box 181, London NW2; tel: 01-459 2440), which have been set up by the parents of affected children in various countries.

COLDS
There is still no cure for the common cold, and treatment is

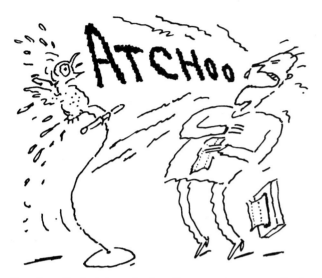

therefore limited to relieving the symptoms, usually by taking aspirin or similar drugs. It's pointless to go to the doctor. Some patients demand penicillin or other antibiotics when they have colds, but to give such drugs would be futile and even possibly harmful. Colds are caused by viruses, and viruses are not killed by antibiotics, or indeed by any other form of therapy available at present (though interferon is showing promise!)

Most people find that taking plenty of fluids helps the misery of a bad cold. Fresh air and exercise are usually better than inactivity in a stuffy room. Alcohol is favoured by many patients, but leaves others feeling worse than before when the effect of the drink wears off. Vitamin C taken in the doses normally stated has been shown scientifically to be quite useless. However, Linus Pauling, the Nobel prize-winner, maintains that enormous doses of the vitamin have an anti-cold effect. At the present time, few doctors agree with this view.

COLIC

This is a word used to describe any gripping pain that 'comes and goes', including the typical pain caused by kidney stones and gall bladder stones. Most commonly, however, colic means the pain associated with painful spasm of the intestines. Most people suffer from this occasionally, usually as part of some minor tummy upset. Frequently the pain goes as soon as the patient has had his bowels open. The most helpful immediate measure is to place a hot water bottle on the abdomen. Do not take aspirin or purges, which may make things worse.

Colic in babies is very common indeed, particularly between the first and third month of life. It usually comes on in the evening, and the baby may scream for several hours. There is no easy answer to this problem, and the parents are often at their wits' end after a few weeks.

However, infantile colic of this type usally ceases altogether when the baby is about three months old. Most such children grow extremely well, so the colic obviously does them no harm. The family GP or the baby clinic doctor will advise as to adjustment of feeds or use of medicines, but unfortunately time is often the only healer.

COLITIS (*See* ULCERATIVE COLITIS.)

COLOSTOMY

An artificial opening for the bowel (colon). Operations involving making a colostomy or an ileostomy (which is very similar to a colostomy) are very widely performed nowadays, for such conditions as DIVERTICULITIS, ULCERATIVE COLITIS, and bowel growths. The aperture is usually made in the lower part of the abdomen. It is covered by special plastic bags, which are, of course, changed frequently. Some adjustment of diet will usually be necessary, but otherwise the patient can lead a perfectly normal life.

Sometimes it is possible to remove the colostomy and restore the bowels to normal when internal healing has taken place. This is what happened in the case of the Pope, who had a 'temporary colostomy' after a would-be assassin's bullet hit his colon.

Anyone who has a colostomy (or who knows he is going to have one) should contact the Colostomy Welfare Group. 38 Ecclestone Sq, London, SW1, for their very valuable help and advice.

COLOUR BLINDNESS

This condition occurs in various forms, but far and away the most frequently encountered is the type in which red and green are confused. This is an inherited condition, present in about 3% of all men, but not in women. Affected people often don't realize they have the defect, which obviously troubles them very little, except if they are working in jobs which require accurate colour differentiation, like lab work or work in the field of fashion. In the UK, it is usually possible for a colour-blind person to drive, because of the fixed position of the lights, but you should declare the condition when applying for a licence.

CONJUNCTIVITIS

Inflammation of the membrane covering the white of the

eye. This may be caused by infection with germs, or by damage due to grit, etc. There is pinkness of the eye, and often some yellow, sticky discharge. If bathing with boric acid lotion is not helpful, consult your doctor, who will probably prescribe antibiotic drops or ointment. A baby with conjunctivitis should always be seen by a doctor.

CONSTIPATION

Up until about 1950, constipation was still widely regarded as rather an important condition which had all sorts of ill-effects on the body. This Victorian attitude is now known to be absolute nonsense—but unfortunately it will probably be several generations before all the public lose the obsession with the bowels that many of them had drummed into them in childhood!

Neither children nor adults *necessarily* have to pass motions every day—many people have a natural rhythm which involves only having the bowels open once or twice a week. This does no harm.

Children should *not* be regularly dosed with laxatives, which may be potentially harmful. Such drugs should be banished from family medicine cabinets. It's significant that they are not usually found in doctors' homes.

If bowel action seems more sluggish than normal, the remedy is usually to eat more roughage, and particularly fruit. Exercise and fresh air are also generally felt to be helpful. Bran is pretty good too.

If, however, you tend to become anxious and worried because of failure to 'perform' regularly, and if you can't convince yourself that it really doesn't matter, then try to stick to very mild laxatives, and use them as sparingly as possible. A suitable preparation is liquid paraffin, but even this should not be employed repeatedly over a period of years.

Warning

The one exception to what has been said above is the case of a middle-aged or elderly person who develops sudden constipation for no apparent reason. This may sometimes be a symptom of serious trouble in the intestines, and should be investigated by a doctor (*not* self-treated with ever-increasing doses of laxatives!).

CORNS

A corn is a local hardening and thickening of the skin, invariably caused by wearing shoes that are too tight. People who go barefoot do not develop corns—as I found when I practised in the tropics! The ideal treatment is probably to throw away every shoe you possess and buy some a size or

two larger! Very few patients take this advice and, as a result, most of them continue to be plagued by corns till their dying day.

Local treatment is best undertaken by a chiropodist, but corn plasters provide useful temporary relief, and will dissolve away the core of an obstinate corn.

Don't cut your own corns, or you may end up with an infected toe.

CORONARY THROMBOSIS

This term literally means a clot (or thrombus) in the arteries supplying the heart. Such an occurrence would cut off the blood supply to part of the heart muscle, and cause a 'heart attack'.

In fact, 'heart attack' is a much better term than 'coronary thrombosis', because very often in such episodes there is no actual clot in the coronary arteries—just a *spasm* which has closed down the artery. However, the words 'coronary thrombosis' are now so well established in the language that they will undoubtedly continue to be used for generations. (Doctors call such attacks 'myocardial infarcts', which not only sounds rather vulgar, but shows that as a profession we're far too prone to using long, incomprehensible words.)

The characteristic symptom of a coronary is sudden, severe, crushing central chest pain, which may run down the left arm. The patient is often shocked, and may collapse.

The immediate treatment is to keep the patient lying flat but comfortable. If he is very pale, with a clammy skin and a very weak pulse, then propping his legs and lower trunk up a foot or two may help. If heartbeat or breathing stop, you may have to give cardiac massage or the 'kiss of life' (*see* FIRST AID TECHNIQUES OF RESUSCITATION in the A–Z of Emergencies).

A coronary is a serious business, and most patients who have one must have a spell in hospital, and have to take things very easily for a month or two thereafter. Once convalescence is over, all normal activities, including work, light exercise, and love-making, can normally be resumed.

Prevention of Coronaries

Coronaries have been on the increase among middle-aged and even quite young men in Western countries for years—except in the USA, where greater attention to health, diet and exercise seems to have at last reduced the death rate.

Factors which lead up to these attacks are *(i)* lack of exercise; *(ii)* being overweight; *(iii)* smoking; *(iv)* heredity; *(v)* diet; and *(vi)* possibly worry and strain. The average man who wants to avoid a coronary can do something about all of these with the exception of heredity: if your father or brother has had a coronary, you may be in line too, so there's added need for precautions.

No one can be certain that he's safe against the virtual epidemic of coronary disease that has swept across the industrialized nations in the last 80 years. The best protection lies in taking sensible exercise most days, in keeping the weight down to average levels, in avoiding smoking at all costs, and (so far as we know) in cutting down on the dietary intake of animal fats (especially milk, butter and fried food generally). Sugar intake should also be kept down. Try to avoid too much stress and strain, and put the cares of the office behind you when you return home in the evening.

Finally, if possible, have your doctor keep an eye on your heart, blood pressure and so on as you go through middle-age.

If from this formidable list of instructions I had to select the most important point of all, I think at the moment it would be exercise. The primitive hunter who runs all day across country looking for animal prey does not get coronaries. The man who sits behind a desk or at the wheel of a car or lorry does (especially if he keeps puffing at a fag!).

You may not be able to run across the desert all day long, but you can walk to the station in the morning and back again in the evening; and you can go for a swim in the lunch-hour or have a work-out at night. And if you choose not to—well, it's your funeral.

COUGH

This is one of the commonest of all symptoms, but self-diagnosis of the cause of a cough isn't easy. Any cough

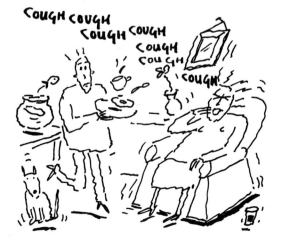

which is present for more than a few days needs treatment by a doctor. Any cough that is present more than two or three weeks needs investigation—at the very least, a chest X-ray.

An X-ray is also essential if blood is coughed up (haemoptysis). This symptom can indicate well over a dozen different conditions of the throat, windpipe, lungs or heart. Some are trivial but others are *serious*, so always go and see your doctor if this happens to you.

CROHN'S DISEASE

'Regional ileitis' is the other name for this fairly common intestinal disease, in which the lining of the bowel becomes inflamed and thickened. Symptoms include recurrent abdominal pain, diarrhoea and bleeding from the rectum. Treatment is usually medical (*i.e.* by drugs) rather than surgical initially, but operation may be necessary. The cause is still unknown.

CROUP

This is the name applied to any condition in which there is partial obstruction of a child's breathing at the level of the throat or the voice-box, *with a resultant crowing noise at each breath.*

Conditions which can cause croup include LARYNGITIS, WHOOPING COUGH, DIPHTHERIA (very rare today) and foreign bodies in the larynx. Until medical aid arrives, sit the child near a steaming kettle (but not too near as the steam will burn)—the moist vapour will ease his breathing. Many such cases are best treated in hospital.

CYSTIC FIBROSIS

Cystic fibrosis is a condition which occurs about once in every 3,000 babies, and which causes a very great deal of distress.

Also known as CF or mucoviscidosis, it's a disease in which the *mucus* produced by certain organs of the body is far thicker and more viscid than normal. The affected organs may include the child's lungs and pancreas.

Because CF is due to inheritance of a faulty gene, there's often a history of another affected child in the family. This may help to give a clue to the diagnosis—which is not always easy.

The disease tends to show itself in one of three ways:
● Recurrent chest infections. The production of thick mucus in the lungs may give the baby or toddler recurring and severe bouts of coughing and wheezing.
● Blockage of the intestines in the newborn. This occurs

because the disease has hit the pancreas—which therefore cannot produce the juices which should digest food.
● Frequent passing of large, pale bowel motions. This again is due to disease of the pancreas.

The *diagnosis* of CF is made by finding unusually high amounts of salt in the child's sweat (mothers often notice that the child tastes abnormally salty).

This is, I'm afraid, a very serious disease. But the outlook has improved quite a bit in recent years. Treatment may include antibiotics to control lung infections; aerosol inhalations; oxygen; physiotherapy; vitamin supplements; and a digestion-promoting powder called pancreatin which helps replace the missing pancreatic juices.

CYSTITIS

This means inflammation of the bladder; but in many cases which are labelled 'cystitis' there is inflammation of the rest of the urinary passages and often of the kidneys too. For this reason, cystitis is not entirely the trivial 'chill' that many people imagine it to be. In recent years, it has become clear that cystitis, unless properly treated, can sometimes have serious consequences on the kidneys (*see* PYELITIS).

The symptoms of cystitis are *pain on passing water* and *a frequent desire to do so*. There is sometimes a little blood in the urine. Quite often, these symptoms follow a woman's first experiences of love-making ('honeymoon cystitis').

As a general rule, cystitis is due to infection by germs which have entered the opening of the urinary passage (the urethra) and made their way up to the bladder.

In women, this passage is very, very short and, of course, very near the rectum—from which most such germs come. This is why cystitis is very common in women, but very rare in men (except those with prostate trouble)—in fact, a man who developed cystitis without apparent reason would need a careful investigation of his urinary system, including X-rays, to see if some structural abnormality was present.

Treatment, if it's to be effective, is slightly complicated. It's certainly not sufficient to go along and ask the doctor for a bottle of medicine, and then forget about the whole thing if the symptoms go off in a couple of days.

Nowadays, the doctor will usually send a specially collected specimen of urine to the lab before he starts treatment—often a 10 day course of antibiotics. The result of this test will (with luck) let him know whether he's got you on the right antibiotic.

Incidentally, until the antibiotic starts working, you can relieve your pain by drinking plenty of fluid, putting a hot water bottle over your bladder, and taking a little bicarbonate of soda.

D

DANDRUFF

This is a trying and very widespread condition. It's *not* as people often imagine, spread from person to person by combs —in fact, it is not caused by germs, and is therefore completely non-infectious. It is related to an over-dryness of the scalp, with consequent scaling of the top layer of skin (*seborrhoea*).

Mild dandruff can usually be kept in check by the regular use of a proprietary 'medicated' shampoo. The word 'medicated' usually indicates that the preparation contains aspirin in liquid form. Some anti-dandruff shampoos contain an antiseptic, though the value of this is doubtful, since, as I've already stressed, the condition is not caused by germs.

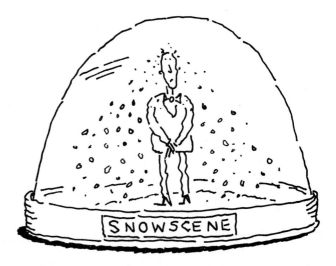

More severe dandruff needs treating by the person's GP, or sometimes by a dermatologist. Difficult cases may never clear up entirely, but can usually be kept well under control. Where dandruff appears in adolescence, there is a tendency to natural improvement, and many patients lose the condition completely by the time they are aged 20 to 25.

DEAFNESS

Deafness is a common complaint which should always be investigated by a doctor. Very often, an elderly person assumes that his increasing hardness of hearing is just an inevitable accompaniment to advancing years. He fails to seek medical advice, and the deafness worsens, with the result that he becomes more and more cut off from those around him.

Many cases of deafness can be greatly helped, and some can be cured. It's surprising how often a person is found to be suffering from nothing more serious than a large accumulation of wax, which can easily be syringed out.

A few cases of deafness (particularly in youngish and middle-aged women) are due to *otosclerosis*—a hardening of the bones in the middle ear. There was little that could be done for this tragically common condition until the 1960s, when a series of brilliant new ear operations were invented. These restore hearing to normal or near-normal levels in the majority of patients with otosclerosis. It was probably this disease that caused Beethoven's deafness.

Even the common nerve deafness of old age can be greatly helped these days by means of modern hearing aids. The best of these are truly remarkable devices so designed as to be almost unnoticeable. If at all possible it's best to obtain one on the recommendation of an ear, nose and throat (ENT) specialist, and not just by sending for a mail-order aid.

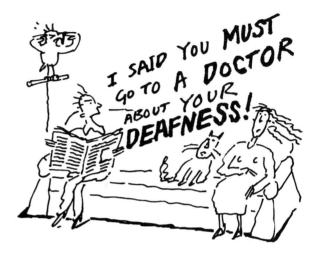

Deafness in Children

CONGENITAL DEAFNESS. Deafness present from birth may be due to the mother acquiring German measles during early pregnancy. Very often, though, the precise cause is not known. Deafness may be total or partial.

An observant mother will sometimes notice by the time the baby is six months old that he is not responding to sound. Other mothers may not notice that anything is wrong until the child is two or three; this is particularly likely to happen where the infant has cleverly learned to interpret the parent's movements and gestures to compensate for the speech it cannot hear.

However, in countries where child health clinics carry out routine examinations of infants, deafness is likely to be picked up by the age of a year. Speech training should start right away. A hearing aid will be provided, and lip-reading instruction will probably be given later on. If these measures are not taken, the child will almost inevitably become backward, and will have immense difficulty in talking properly. Intensive and early treatment gives excellent results, however, and many congenitally deaf children go on to lead happy, full and useful lives.

DEAFNESS LATER IN CHILDHOOD. *Slight* deafness during an attack of earache or a bout of catarrh is common, but, if the deafness persists for more than a week or so, investigation may well be necessary. It has been shown that quite a proportion of children who have apparently recovered from an attack of earache are left with some degree of deafness afterwards. Some ENT specialists believe that all children should have audiograms (special hearing tests) after a bout of earache, but at the moment this doesn't seem to be remotely practicable, since there are just so many kids with earache.

The best course seems to be to make rough tests of the child's hearing a few weeks after the attack. Can he hear the ticking of a watch held against the ear? Can he hear words whispered across the room? (Remember to make sure the child is not lip-reading.) If there is any doubt whatever about the results of these rough tests, take the child back to your doctor.

DEGENERATIVE JOINT DISEASE (DJD) (*See* **Osteoarthritis** under ARTHRITIS.)

DEMENTIA (*See* BRAIN in A–Z of Parts of the Body.)

DEPRESSION

This is a very, very widespread form of psychological illness—so widespread that in the last few years it has become commonplace for general practitioners to see as many as a dozen new cases each week.

Many of these patients have short illnesses, in which the

depression persists only for a matter of a couple of weeks or months. In other cases, depression is a recurrent phenomenon, which troubles the victim intermittently throughout life. In either instance, modern treatment can help greatly.

Symptoms

The chief symptoms of depression include feelings of misery, guilt and worthlessness. Life tends to seem futile and colourless. In some patients, the main complaints are of weakness, tiredness, lack of energy, inability to cope, failure of sexual drive, persistent vague aches and pains, dizziness, muzziness, light-headedness and so on.

In the great majority of cases, *there is a characteristic disturbance of sleep rhythm.* Usually the patient either cannot get off to sleep at night, or else wakes up in the early hours of the morning and lies brooding for hours. Some sufferers sleep fitfully all night, dream a great deal, and wake up exhausted.

In many cases of depression there is a clear cause for the patient's reaction—commonly, of course, the death of a loved one. Other precipitating factors include pregnancy and childbirth (especially when unwanted), influenza, and retirement or redundancy. The outlook is generally better in these cases where the depression is a clear reaction to some external event.

Treatment

The first step on the road to recovery is, of course, to see the doctor, rather than try to bottle the symptoms up. Just talking about their feelings makes many patients feel rather better. Friends and relatives should encourage them to talk too, and try to be understanding of their fluctuations in mood. *Any talk of suicide should always be taken seriously.* If a person has no one he or she feels able to talk to, the Samaritans are at the other end of a phone 24 hours a day, specially to listen to people's troubles in order to help them —but not to give advice. Look in the phone book for their number. Most people who kill themselves have mentioned to relatives, friends or sometimes their doctor that they are considering the idea. All too often, they are laughed at or told to pull themselves together—with tragic results.

Apart from listening to the patient's troubles, the doctor will nowadays usually prescribe antidepressant tablets— which are NOT the same as tranquillisers. These produce a valuable elevation in mood, but it may take 10 days or more before an improvement is obtained. Some changing around of tablets may be needed before a suitable drug is found.

In more severe cases, the doctor will often refer the patient to a psychiatrist, who can provide other forms of treatment, sometimes including ECT (electroconvulsive therapy). Although this sounds alarming, it is quite painless, being carried out under general anaesthesia, usually as an outpatient. It gives particularly good results in 'involutional melancholia', the form of depression so often seen in men about the age of retirement. In such cases, it will frequently terminate the depressive episode and restore the patient completely to normal health. But it can affect the memory.

DIABETES INSIPIDUS

Nothing to do with 'ordinary' diabetes (or DIABETES MELLITUS—see below). This is a rare condition of the pituitary gland (located at the base of the brain). Deficiency of one of the pituitary hormones makes the patient pass vast quantities of water—say, 20 litres (approx 35.2 pints) a day! Treatment is with a pituitary hormone given by injection or as a nasal 'snuff'.

DIABETES MELLITUS

This is 'ordinary' or 'sugar' diabetes.

Diabetes is one of the most common diseases known to man, and its frequency appears to be increasing. This is probably because of the marked tendency in Western society for people to overeat and to be overweight.

What is Diabetes?

To understand diabetes, you've first got to understand how the body is fuelled. Just as a car needs petrol, the body needs glucose, which is a form of sugar. This doesn't have to be taken as glucose tablets or powder by mouth—any carbohydrate (*i.e.* starchy or sugary) food will be rapidly broken down by the digestive system, and turned into glucose, which will then circulate in the blood and be 'burned' in the tissues to provide energy.

However, the blood glucose (or blood sugar, as it is often called) will not 'burn' unless insulin is present. Insulin is a chemical manufactured in the pancreas, a gland located just under the stomach. With diabetes, something has gone badly wrong with this organ.

We still don't fully understand what this change is but basically there is not enough insulin, and therefore too much sugar circulating in the bloodstream.

The excess sugar spills over into the urine, where it can be detected by a simple test. Symptoms which are associated with the elevated blood sugar level include vomiting, loss of weight, exhaustion, great thirst, and the passing of large quantities of urine.

In the younger diabetic, these symptoms are usually very severe at the onset of the disease. They are often accompanied by drowsiness, which, if untreated over a period of days, may progress to diabetic coma—a very serious medical emergency.

Treatment

YOUNGER DIABETICS. Such patients usually need a strict diet, and daily insulin injections all their lives to keep the blood sugar down to reasonable levels. (However, my colleague Dr Gerry Humphreys and I found that young West Indian diabetics often didn't need insulin.)

If several injections are missed, or if insufficient insulin is being given, or if some other illness (*e.g.* an infection) upsets the balance, then the blood sugar may get out of control again, and the patient slip into diabetic coma.

The sensible diabetic, however, will have early warning that something is going wrong, because his morning urine test (or blood test—for which some patients now have facilities) will usually have shown heavy concentration of sugar over a period of two or three days.

It is very important for diabetics to do these simple daily tests themselves, and to keep a record of the results. This can be shown to the doctor at each visit. If the patient is unlucky enough to be found unconscious, the record will be an invaluable guide as to what has been going on, and whether diabetic coma is present.

In fact, the great majority of cases of unconsciousness among diabetics are due *not* to too much sugar (diabetic coma) but to too little. Such attacks are called 'insulin reactions', or 'hypos'. They occur when the patient is having too much insulin, or too little carbohydrate food to balance it. The most recent urine test will usually have been sugar-free. The attacks come on suddenly, often when a meal is late, and usually start with a short period of weakness and mental confusion. Diabetics' relatives rapidly learn to recognise these symptoms and to apply the remedy, which is to give sugar by mouth as fast as possible.

The occurrence of 'hypos' is usually an indication that the dose of insulin should be slightly reduced.

DIABETICS WHO DON'T NEED INSULIN. For simplicity (and to stress that diabetes is a question of balance between sugar on the one hand, and insulin on the other) we've only dealt so far with 'insulin-dependent' diabetics, who usually acquire the disease fairly early in life.

Most diabetics, however, do *not* require injections of insulin, but can manage with a strict low-carbohydrate diet, often supplemented by anti-diabetic tablets. These patients are usually overweight, and they tend to develop the disease in later life. The basic principles of control are exactly the same for them as for the 'insulin-dependent' diabetics,

but there is usually virtually no risk of the blood sugar ever rising so high as to put the patient into diabetic coma. There is, however, a risk of 'hypos' if the patient is taking too large a dose of antidiabetic tablets.

GENERAL: The best course for any diabetic lies in taking his treatment with strict regularity, keeping to his diet, testing the urine (or blood, if possible) for sugar each day, and seeing the doctor regularly for adjustment of therapy. Attending a hospital clinic which specializes in diabetes is usually an advantage.

DIARRHOEA

Acute diarrhoea

Attacks of diarrhoea in adults or in older children are usually due to a 'bug'—*i.e.* a minor bowel infection.

Diarrhoea of this type tends to 'go round' families or schools in mini-epidemics. It is also very common on holidays —as 'traveller's tummy' or 'gyppy tummy'. Useful remedies are kaolin mixture or codeine phosphate tablets.

Some cases of diarrhoea, particularly when travelling, are probably caused by the effect of unusual and highly spiced foods. The immediate treatment is the same—take kaolin or coedine phosphate, and stick to fluids only for at least 24 hours.

In any case of acute diarrhoea, it is essential to take preventive measures to stop possible spread of germs from person to person. The patient should not be allowed to touch other people's food. Hands should be washed before meals, before cooking and (very important) after visiting the toilet. On camping, boating or caravanning holidays, great care should be taken in disposal of excreta.

Warning: beware of severe diarrhoea in a baby, as it can be very serious. Always check with a doctor (see below).

Chronic Diarrhoea

Diarrhoea lasting more than a week or two should always be investigated by a doctor. There are many conditions which can cause this symptom, ranging from the trivial (such as a mild anxiety state) to the severe (such as ulcerative colitis). A barium enema X-ray is sometimes helpful in diagnosis. Diarrhoea after returning from foreign parts may well turn out to be due to some tropical bug.

Diarrhoea in Babies

This is a common symptom, and if it's slight, it's of little significance. But if it persists it is best dealt with by the family doctor. Many babies have a loose bowel action after every feed, and continue to do so for the first six months of life. In others, diarrhoea is simply a reaction to too much sugar in the feed. In a very small proportion of children, it may indicate some important underlying disorder such as coeliac disease (*see* COELIAC DISEASE).

SEVERE DIARRHOEA IN BABIES: An acute attack of violent diarrhoea with repeated passage of watery stools is best regarded as being infectious, and the mother must take extreme care not to spread the germs to other members of the family. Note the hygienic measures outlined above for the prevention of spread of adult diarrhoea; in addition, the hands should be washed very carefully after changing nappies. Advice should be sought from a doctor, though he may not necessarily have to see the child immediately.

A useful plan for emergency treatment is as follows: take the baby completely off milk and solids, and instead give him as much boiled water as he will take. To each pint of boiled water, add a teaspoonful of sugar and a tiny pinch of salt. Alternatively, a commercial fluid replacement product (Dioralyte) is now available.

Warning: if a baby who has severe diarrhoea appears weak and lifeless, with a dry skin, hollow eyes and a sunken fontanelle (the soft spot on top of the head), he is in extreme danger. If you cannot contact a doctor, get the baby to hospital at once.

DIPHTHERIA

This is a dangerous infection which used to be very common in childhood, and which once killed many young babies. Thanks to the introduction of immunization diphtheria is now rare, but in the last few years the incidence has been rising very slightly. This is because parents no longer regard the disease as a serious risk, and many don't have their babies immunized with 'triple' vaccine (which protects against diphtheria, WHOOPING COUGH, and TETANUS).

Diphtheria can take many forms, but the commonest features are fever, sore throat, loss of appetite and vomiting. These symptoms are accompanied by the formation of a pearly-grey membrane at the back of the throat, which can usually be seen when the child's mouth is open. The membrane may choke the child to death if medical aid is not obtained rapidly. So make sure your child has the jab!

If you have decided that you don't want the whooping cough part of the jab, you can ask for the 'double' jab, which just protects against diphtheria and lockjaw.

DISC, SLIPPED (*See* BACKACHE.)

DISLOCATIONS

It's usually fairly easy to tell by appearance that a joint—

for instance, a finger joint—has been dislocated. Bear in mind that a fracture may also have occurred. Do not interfere or try to correct the dislocation yourself. Try to immobilize the affected limb by gently bandaging it to a splint, and get the patient to hospital, where he can be X-rayed and have the injury properly dealt with.

The only exception to this is recurrent dislocation of the shoulder joint. Patients who have suffered this dislocation repeatedly are often adept at replacing the joint themselves, and there's no reason why they should not do so. It is often possible to cure this tendency to recurrent dislocation by means of an operation on the joint.

DIVERTICULAR DISEASE

In about one in 10 of all middle-aged and elderly people, small pouches called 'diverticula' form in the lower bowel, usually just above the rectum. It's widely believed that the development of these pouches is related to the low-fibre type of diet eaten by Western Man, though this is hard to prove.

In many people these pouches cause no symptoms, and they are only discovered incidentally (for instance, during an operation for some other condition). If the pouches become inflamed, however, diverticulitis is said to be present. Common symptoms are pain in the lower left side of the abdomen (either cramps or tenderness to touch), fever, bowel disturbances and bleeding from the rectum.

Careful investigation is necessary. The diagnosis can be made with certainty during surgery or by a barium enema X-ray. Treatment is a complicated business, I'm afraid. Operation may be necessary to remove the diseased bowel— but special 'bowel antibiotics' and a high fibre diet may be sufficient.

DIZZINESS

The word 'dizziness' really means two things. Some people who complain of the symptom mean that the room seems to be spinning around them, just as it would if they turned rapidly in circles. This type of dizziness is known as 'vertigo'. (*See* VERTIGO.)

Much more often, however, people mean simply that they feel weak, faint, or light-headed.

Such symptoms can be due to a variety of causes, many of which are quite trivial (for instance, *postural* dizziness, which is characterized by faint feelings after standing up suddenly). Others (for instance, severe anaemia) may require prompt treatment. The best course is to consult the family doctor, who will usually be able to sort out the cause of the dizziness.

DREAMS

All human beings dream, although not everyone recalls their dreams in the morning. Laboratory experiments show that dreaming occurs for a total of about two hours every night, broken up into half a dozen separate spells averaging around 20 minutes each. During these spells, the eyeballs can be seen to move rapidly from side to side.

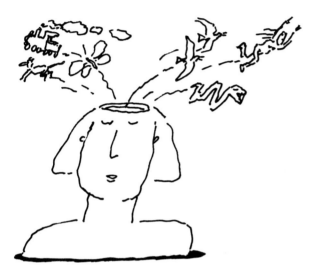

Dreams often alarm people by their content, but in fact they are a necessity to healthy mental life, since they enable a person to 'act out' all the suppressed urges of the day. This is why staid and respectable people often find themselves behaving in the most bizarre and even sexy fashion in their dreams!

Some patients find violent or sexually charged dreams very hard to cope with, and in such circumstances it is probably best to chat with the family doctor, who may be able to help resolve underlying conflicts and provide reassurance.

A great deal has been written in the past about the psycho-sexual symbolism of dreams. It's certainly true that people do tend to express deep sexual conflicts in 'censored' or symbolic terms—the classic example being the frustrated woman who sees in her dreams the phallic symbol of a steeple. In these permissive days, however, it does seem that patients no longer seem to feel quite the same need to express sexuality in this 'hidden' way, and symbolic dreaming of this type is possibly rather less common than it was in Freud's day. On the other hand, persistent dreaming about a particular object or situation may have quite simple symbolic explanation, which will help to resolve some inner conflict.

Nightmares are probably universal. Traditionally, they are said to be made worse by dietary indiscretions (the 'cheese for supper' theory), but they're much more likely to be related to mental stress and strain. Nightmares are particularly likely to occur when the effect of a sleeping pill (or of alcohol) is wearing off.

'Wet dreams' are erotic dreams accompanied by a sexual climax. They are often a source of anxiety to boys who have not been forewarned about them. It is important to realize that these dreams are a normal part of growing up, occurring in virtually every teenage boy (and in many adult males as well, though with lesser frequency).

DROPSY

Dropsy means an unusual accumulation of fluid in the body tissues. Fluid collecting in the body cavities (for instance, in the abdomen) is called *ascites*; this kind of dropsy is usually due to liver or heart trouble.

Fluid collecting in the tissues is called 'oedema' or (if you're American) 'edema'. It tends to accumulate around the ankles, and sometimes below the eyes. The causes of this symptom are many, and include kidney, liver and heart disease, and toxaemia of pregnancy (*see* PREGNANCY).

DRUGS—ABUSE AND ADDICTION (*See* ALCOHOL, AMPHETAMINES, ASPIRIN, BARBITURATES, CANNABIS, HEROIN, MANDRAX, TOBACCO.)

DUODENAL ULCER (*See* ULCERS.)

DYSPEPSIA (*See* INDIGESTION.)

EARACHE

This trying condition is very common in childhood but rare in adults. It is caused by germs spreading from the throat or nose up the tube which leads to the ear. Very often, the child has had a slight cold for a few days prior to the onset of the pain. The aching is intense, and is accompanied by a fever, with the temperature usually being about 101°F (38.3°C) or more.

The first consideration is *relief of pain*: give the child some aspirin in fairly generous dosage (but don't exceed that stated on the bottle) and let him hold a hot water bottle (wrapped in a cloth) over his ear. Use the measures outlined under TEMPERATURE to keep him cool.

Talk to your doctor. He should be consulted within a matter of a few hours if possible. The child will be treated with a course of antibiotics, which may have to be continued for 10 days or so.

It's most important to be on the watch for deafness after a bout of earache. It's advisable for parents to check whether the child can hear sounds such as whispered speech or the ticking of a watch at an interval of, say, one month after the illness. If there is any doubt at all, take the kiddy back to his doctor who will, if necessary, recommend specialist investigation and treatment. (*See also* DEAFNESS.)

ECTOPIC PREGNANCY

This means pregnancy occurring outside the normal situation (*i.e.* the womb). In the great majority of such cases, the fertilised egg lodges in the Fallopian tube (which connects the ovary to the womb). Where this happens there is no possibility that the baby can be born.

In fact, it usually becomes apparent that something is wrong not long after the first period is missed. The symptoms vary a good deal, but usually the woman experiences quite severe pain low down in the abdomen, on either the right or the left side, depending on which tube is involved. Sometimes the pain is accompanied by giddiness. Within a few hours there is usually vaginal bleeding, though this may be slight.

In some cases of ectopic pregnancy there is severe bleeding inside the abdomen. If this happens, the patient collapses and is pale, shocked and gasping for breath. She *must* be got to hospital immediately.

The only treatment for ectopic pregnancy is to remove the foetus by surgical operation. Usually the Fallopian tube has to be taken away as well. This doesn't mean that the patient is now sterile, however; if the other tube is healthy, there is no reason why she should not have children in the future.

Ectopic pregnancies are probably commoner in women who are using the IUD—and possibly in women who are on the mini-Pill.

ECZEMA

This is a very common skin condition—or rather group of conditions, because there are really a number of eczematous disorders. Some people suffer from small patches of eczema only once or twice during their lives; others are plagued by recurrent episodes of *eczematous dermatitis*. Many babies suffer from 'infantile eczema', which is usually (not always) mild and clears up entirely in the first few years of life. A few infants go on having eczema throughout childhood, and some 'exchange' it for asthma as they grow older.

Recent research indicates that some babies develop eczema because they are allergic to cow's milk. So if your family is an allergy-prone one, you should try particularly hard to breast-feed rather than bottle-feed your babies.

In some cases of eczema, there is a strong hereditary element, and in others there isn't. Some people find that their eczema gets much worse when they are under stress, but in other patients there is no relationship to psychological strain.

The word 'eczema', then, can mean many things, and it's not surprising that doctors find difficulty even in agreeing on a definition. Fortunately, methods of treatment of all kinds of eczema have greatly improved in recent years, especially with the introduction of steroid preparations to soothe inflamed skin. In general, it's best to keep the skin as dry as possible (soap, water and detergents being harmful factors), but the patient's GP (or dermatologist) will advise on the best regime. This advice should be followed to the letter—a few people think that just one or two applications of a 'wonder drug' ought to be enough to clear up their skin, but this is very rarely so. Patience is often as important as medication!

Very important: it is now sometimes possible to clear up eczema by cutting some item out of the diet. Ask your dermatologist for details of how to do this.

EMISSIONS, NOCTURNAL (*See* **Wet Dreams**, under DREAMS.)

EMPHYSEMA

This is a chest disease in which there is distortion and destruction of the tissues that make up the lungs. Emphysema mainly occurs in combination with either chronic bronchitis (*see* BRONCHITIS) or asthma (*see* ASTHMA). Occasionally, it follows pneumoconiosis (*see* PNEUMOCONIOSIS). The main feature is severe and increasing breathlessness, in addition to the symptoms of either bronchitis or asthma. Treatment involves absolute avoidance of cigarettes, use of antibiotics when infection of the chest occurs, breathing exercises from a physiotherapist, and correction of any obesity.

ENDOMETRIOSIS

This is a fairly common gynaecological condition, occurring mainly between the ages of 25 and 45. Its characteristic feature is that tissue which normally forms the lining of the womb (endometrial tissue) turns up in abnormal situations, *e.g.* in the navel, in the appendix, in operation scars, in the bowel, and (more commonly) in the ovaries, in the wall of the vagina and in the muscular wall of the womb.

Now, this endometrial tissue responds to female hormones in exactly the same way as normal womb lining does—in other words, it swells up and bleeds at period times. The swelling process may cause considerable pain.

A story of odd pain in various sites occurring during menstruation is suspicious of endometriosis. There may also be pain with intercourse, and often infertility (due to endometriosis of the tubes or ovaries). Diagnosis is made by operation—or by the newish technique of laparoscopy in which the internal organs are inspected with a slim, telescope-like device. Treatment is by surgery or hormone therapy, though irradiation is sometimes helpful. The Pill has turned out to be a useful anti-endometriosis treatment.

ENTERITIS (*See* GASTRO-ENTERITIS.)

ENURESIS (*See* BED-WETTING.)

EPILEPTIC DISORDERS

There's no single disease which can properly be called 'epilepsy'. But there are a wide range of different conditions which have one feature in common. *That feature is a transient episode of disordered brain function during which an abnormal electrical discharge takes place within the central nervous system.* Epileptic disorders are, therefore, no more than a manifestation of a sudden surge of nervous activity—in some ways rather like a gross exaggeration of a sneeze.

Over the centuries, there has, unhappily, been a good deal of prejudice among ignorant people against anyone who suffered from an epileptic disorder. This is mainly because a convulsion can be quite a frightening sight for a person who does not understand its nature—in fact, people used to think that fits indicated possession by demons!

These old ideas die hard, but attitudes are at last changing, and most sensible people now recognize that an epileptic disorder is an illness like any other. Throughout the world there are literally tens of millions of people suffering from some form of epileptic attacks. A very large number of them have fits only rarely, and are able to lead perfectly normal and healthy lives. Many of these people are of high intelligence—which is not surprising when one considers that such men as Socrates, Julius Caesar, Byron, Handel, Dante, Dostoyevsky and Alexander the Great all suffered from fits. It seems manifestly unfair, therefore, that society should continue to attach any stigma whatever to these illnesses. Happily, public awareness that certain well-known sportsmen (for instance, a recent England cricket captain) have epilepsy is beginning to alter these silly prejudices.

Types of Epileptic Disorder

INFANTILE CONVULSIONS. These convulsions are very common indeed. They are usually provoked by a feverish illness, such as a cold or tonsilitis. Most (but not all) affected children have no further fits after the age of five. (*See* CONVULSIONS.)

PETIT MAL. This disorder is very common in childhood, but rare in adults. The child suddenly stares into space and pays no attention to anything around him. After a few seconds he recovers and goes on with what he was doing as if nothing had happened. Literally hundreds of such attacks may occur every day. There's a great tendency for this illness to get better as the child gets older.

GRAND MAL. This is the term for a generalized convulsion. The patient loses consciousness and falls to the ground. His arms and legs twitch, and his teeth are clenched. After a variable period of time, lasting anything between half a minute and five minutes, he slowly recovers consciousness, but he will usually feel poorly for some hours afterwards, and should be given the chance to lie down and go to sleep for a while.

This is the common type of major fit seen in most seizure-prone adults (and in many children). *First aid treatment* should be limited to ensuring the patient does not injure himself (*e.g.* by rolling onto a fire). Prising the teeth apart is dangerous, but if the patient's mouth chances to open, a handkerchief may be slipped between the jaws to prevent biting of the tongue. Similarly, false teeth may be removed if the opportunity arises.

It is usually best to keep the patient lying on his side as he recovers. There is normally no need to call an ambulance or a doctor unless the fit shows no signs of terminating after three minutes or so.

Grand mal fits in children show a heartening tendency to become less frequent as the youngster gets older.

FITS STARTING IN LATER LIFE. These should never simply be written off as 'due to epilepsy', but investigated carefully. Possible causes include past head injury, cerebral tumour, drug addiction (particularly withdrawal of barbiturates or of alcohol in an addicted person), and minor strokes.

OTHER TYPES OF FIT. There are many other types of convulsive disorder, particularly in childhood, but their diagnosis and management are really too complex to be discussed here. Some of them are associated with severe brain injury at or before birth.

Treatment

Anyone who has had a fit (with the exception of an infant who has had only a single feverish convulsion) should have an electroencephalogram (EEG), or electrical test of the activity of the brain waves. This is often a considerable help to diagnosis and therapy.

An increasing range of drugs are available for the suppression of attacks, but it is essential to realize that these are only effective *if they are taken regularly*. Missing a dose or allowing the tablets to run out will very possibly lead to fresh attacks.

The drugs used do have important side-effects, which is one reason why the patient should be seen regularly by his GP and, from time to time, by a specialist as well. Children should be seen by the pediatrician at quite frequent intervals, since correct adjustment of the dose of drugs may be very difficult—too much too often makes the child unsteady on his feet and can lead to behaviour problems.

A big advance in recent years has been the development of tests to measure the blood levels of the anti-epileptic drugs. Previously, a lot of people were wandering round with far too high drug levels—which made them drowsy, confused or irritable. Everyone with epilepsy should have these levels checked occasionally.

As I've said above, as a child gets older, there's often a tendency for his illness to improve, and fits may sometimes cease altogether. If so, the drugs can usually be tailed off carefully under the guidance of the specialist. Where fits persist into adulthood, however, the hospital should give help regarding employment and social problems. The British Epilepsy Association (Bigshotte, Crowthorne, Berks, tel: Crowthorne 3122) operates advice services which may be of considerable assistance to both children and adults suffering from this group of illnesses.

ERYSIPELAS

This is a skin inflammation, caused by a germ called the streptococcus, which is present in many people's throats and noses. The skin becomes reddened and hot, and feels hard to the touch. There is often fever, headache and vomiting. The infection usually responds to antibiotic treatment.

Erysipelas used at one time to be quite a common condition, with a death rate of about 15%. Nowadays, it's not often encountered, and easily treated with antibiotics.

EYE DISORDERS (*See* CATARACTS, COLOUR BLINDNESS, CONJUNCTIVITIS, GLAUCOMA, STYES.)

F

FATNESS

At least a third of all people in Western countries carry more weight than is good for them, but surprisingly few are willing to admit that they are fat! People with vast paunches or doughy hips talk about 'having just a little middle-aged spread', or 'being well covered'. They almost invariably deny that they ever eat much (which *may* be true), and attribute their condition to glands, heredity, or advancing years.

The plain fact is that every pound of excess weight shortens the life expectancy slightly—try getting an insurance company to give you a life insurance policy at normal rates if you are obese!

Furthermore, fat comes from one source and one source only—food. It cannot, as so many seem to think, be formed out of thin air, or manifest itself in some strange supernatural fashion. Admittedly, some people 'burn' food less well than normal—probably because of a lack of certain brown fat cells in their bodies. But if you eat little and you are still fat, then the only answer is to eat even less! Few people will face up to this uncomfortable fact, which is why so-called 'slimming clinics' are able to make vast sums of money out of gullible folk who can be persuaded that impressive-looking machines and strange garments will make them lose weight.

Nor, unfortunately, is a small amount of exercise a great deal of help. Exercise is certainly very good for the health in other ways, but it only burns up a relatively small quantity of food. Some researchers have calculated that you would need to walk 30 miles in order to burn up a pound of fat. (The *temporary* weight loss after violent exercise is due entirely to the amount of water lost in sweating; it is invariably replaced within a matter of hours.)

On the other hand, it's often forgotten that REGULAR and FAIRLY ENERGETIC exercise must burn up at least *some* fat over a long period of time. Thus, if you blanch at the thought of walking 30 miles to burn up a pound of fat, bear in mind that a two-mile walk every day tots up to almost 30 miles a fortnight. So walking two miles a day would burn up a pound of fat every two weeks—or 26 pounds a year!

But losing weight is almost entirely a matter of great will-power. Some patients do find that their appetites are suppressed by certain drugs, but many others do not. And, unfortunately, drugs do have side effects: some even cause addiction.

Dieting

What foods should you avoid? It is really best if you can get a calorie-controlled diet sheet (*e.g.* 800, 1,000, or 1,200 calories) from your doctor, particularly as there are some people who should not embark blindly on a slimming diet without medical advice.

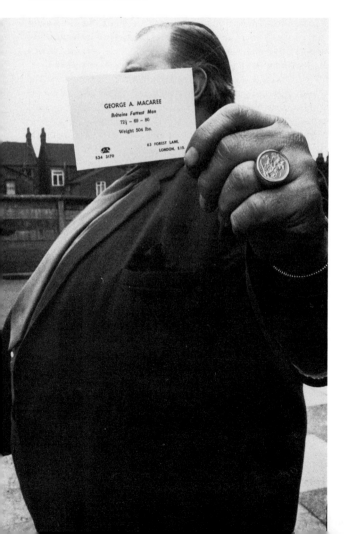

In general, however, the determined slimmer should have none of the following: potatoes, sugar, cake, pastry, biscuits, sweets, puddings, soft drinks, jam, alcohol—*and, above all, fatty foods.* Fat contains TWICE the calories of other foods. The slimmer should beware of the following: butter or margarine, cheese and milk.

On the other hand, she or he can have plenty of the following: green vegetables, tomatoes, grapefruit and all other fairly low sugar content fruits, lean meat, fish, tea, coffee, and beef extract drinks.

Some patients find that eating special products containing methyl cellulose is helpful, since this substance expands in the stomach and produces a feeling of fullness. Most people do not find such 'foods' much use, however.

'Slimming foods' in general should be viewed with caution. They are usually expensive, and they are only 'slimming' in the sense that they usually contain slightly less calories than the equivalent 'ordinary' food. A recent survey showed that some types of so-called slimming bread had more calories than ordinary bread. Where anything to do with slimming is concerned, *caveat emptor*—let the buyer beware!

FEVER (*See* TEMPERATURE.)

FIBROIDS
These are benign swellings which occur within the muscular wall of the womb. They usually develop between the age of thirty and the time of the change of life, and are more common in women who have not had any children. Their cause is not known.

Very often fibroids do not produce symptoms, and don't require any treatment. They may, however, cause heavy or prolonged periods, with resulting anaemia. Other possible symptoms include pain and discharge. Sometimes, the patient's only symptom is a large swelling low down in the abdomen.

Small symptomless fibroids do not need therapy. Larger fibroids are usually removed surgically. It's sometimes possible to shell the fibroids out from the wall of the womb, but more often hysterectomy (*see* HYSTERECTOMY) is necessary.

FIBROSITIS
This is a popular term—but I'm afraid it doesn't really mean anything and it's no longer used in medicine! Most people employ it to mean approximately the same thing as 'rheumatism'. (*See* RHEUMATISM.)

Fat may be famous—but it's not healthy.

FLAT FOOT

The foot is an arched structure, which is why, when a child with healthy feet gets out of the bath, the footprints he leaves on the bathroom floor show that most of the sole of his foot is off the ground. Where this is not so, the foot is referred to as being flat.

There are in fact two basic types of flat foot—*pes planus* and *pes valgus*. Pes planus is less common, and is often associated with some minor structural abnormality of the bones of the foot. In pes valgus there is no structural abnormality, but the foot rolls inwards when bearing weight due to laxity of the muscles and ligaments of the lower part of the leg.

The first treatment used is often an intensive course of exercise. An arch support made of moulded leather or a plastic heel seat may prove of value but it is essential that such supports are worn all day long. Surgical treatment is occasionally helpful. I must stress that many children with mild flat foot will get better without any treatment other than a periodic check-up by the doctor, and plenty of encouragement to run about.

FLEA BITES

Flea infestation is fortunately less common than it used to be though cat fleas have become a nuisance in Britain in recent years! In warm parts of the world, fleas may sometimes carry diseases such as plague or typhus. Even the most scrupulously clean people may sometimes be bitten by these creatures, and if this occurs, all bedding and clothing should be carefully laundered. The patient's doctor may suggest dusting the skin and the seams of clothing with DDT powder.

Where cat fleas are attacking your family, get your poor old puss intensively treated with a spray from the vet. You may have to treat furniture and carpets too.

FLOODING (*See* VAGINA in the A–Z of Parts of the Body.)

FOOD POISONING

This may be due to germs (or germ toxins) in food, to toxic chemicals, or to allergy to food. It causes diarrhoea and vomiting.

Germs

The most common type of food poisoning is due to germs. *Staphylococci* are the germs found in boils and 'spots', and in many people's noses. They produce a toxin (poison) which is quite unaffected by cooking or even boiling. If this toxin gets into food, anyone who eats it will develop nausea, vomiting, colicky abdominal pains, and diarrhoea, all within a few hours. The attack does not last long, and can usually be treated by the patient's doctor at home. This type of food poisoning would be less common if people took more care about hygiene when preparing food—particularly washing their hands!

Salmonella are germs which produce similar symptoms to the above, but about 24–48 hours after eating infected food. The illness may be quite severe and last several days. A laboratory test on the stools will identify the germ and let the doctor know what antibiotic to use.

This type of food poisoning may be caused by contaminated meat (especially tinned meat and sausages). Duck's eggs and shellfish may also be responsible. Seemingly healthy 'carriers' of Salmonella germs can cause attacks of food poisoning in other people if they do not wash their hands properly after visiting the toilet and before preparing food.

Viruses may also cause food poisoning. These are also passed on by faulty hygiene.

Other Types of Food Poisoning

Chemical food poisoning is rare—the most important variety is probably fungus poisoning (*see* TOADSTOOL POISONING).

Allergy to food or food additives may produce a wide variety of symptoms, as well as diarrhoea and vomiting. There may be eczema, urticaria ('hives') on the skin, and asthma attacks. Desensitization treatment, by means of

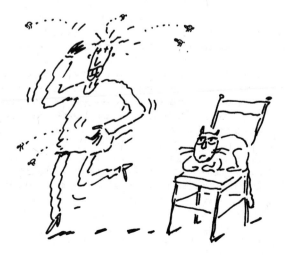

injections of very small quantities of the food protein involved, is sometimes attempted. But it's best to try to find out what the 'danger' food is—and cut it out of your diet.

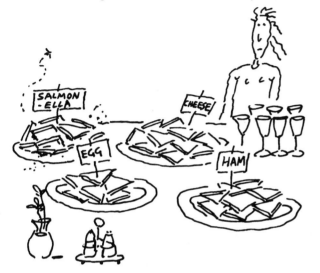

G

GASTRIC ULCER (*See* ULCERS.)

GASTRITIS

This word just means inflammation of the stomach. The features are vomiting and sometimes tenderness in the upper part of the abdomen. If retching is violent or repeated, blood may be brought up. If this happens, you should consult a doctor.

Gastritis is usually due to an infection of the digestive tract, but is sometimes caused by over-indulgence in alcohol or aspirin. It is often associated with inflammation of the intestines as well as the stomach, in which case the condition is known as gastro-enteritis. For treatment, see under GASTRO-ENTERITIS.

GASTRO-ENTERITIS

Inflammation of the stomach and intestinal tract. The features are those of gastritis (see GASTRITIS) together with diarrhoea and often colicky pain low down in the abdomen.

The cause of gastro-enteritis is usually infection by a germ. So it follows that most cases could be avoided by good hygiene in the home and in food preparation, as with preventing the spread of diarrhoea. Preventing the spread of infection is discussed under the heading DIARRHOEA.

Treatment

If vomiting is very troublesome, any medicine taken by mouth is likely to be brought straight back. If the patient can swallow a soothing preparation such as magnesium trisilicate and keep it down, then well and good. Most 'tummy upsets' do not really need any medication, however, and the patient will get better if he stays on fluids only for 24 hours or so. It is often best to begin with sips of water and progress, after perhaps 12 hours, to milk or fruit juice.

If diarrhoea is severe, kaolin mixture will prove helpful once the patient can keep things down. After an attack of gastro-enteritis, it's best to stick to small helpings of light meals for a week or so. Aspirin, alcohol and spicy foods should be avoided, since they may irritate the stomach. (*See also* FOOD POISONING.)

GERMAN MEASLES (RUBELLA)

This is a common infectious disease caused by a virus. It has nothing to do with ordinary measles.

Features

The incubation period is 12–21 days. The features of the condition vary a great deal, so that the disease is often far more difficult to diagnose with certainty than most people imagine! The commonest symptoms are: first, a day or two of general ill-health, with perhaps a slight sore throat, and then the development of a fine, blotchy, pink rash over the face, neck, and trunk. The temperature is slightly raised, and there is very often enlargement of the glands at the back of the neck.

In a clear cut case, the only treatment required is bed rest for a day or two, with plenty of fluids and perhaps a little aspirin if the throat is sore. The child should be kept at home until the doctor says he can go out. He *must* be kept away from any expectant mothers until at least two weeks after the onset of the symptoms.

Expectant Mothers

The reason for this is that there is great danger that German measles in a pregnant woman will cause her baby to be born malformed. The risk is greatest in the first three months of pregnancy, but there may be some slight danger even at five months. The mother may never even have shown the rash or the other features of the disease. An affected child may have severe abnormalities of the heart or the ears, or may be born blind. For this reason, most gynaecologists are willing to terminate a pregnancy where the mother is believed to have had German measles.

It used to be the practice to give injections of gamma globulin (which contains protective antibodies) to mothers who had been exposed to rubella. Recent work suggests that this did not protect babies after all.

An expectant mother in this position can, however, have a blood test to determine whether she is already immune to German measles. If she is (as 80% of women are), then she has nothing to worry about. If she is not, then she can have the test repeated shortly afterwards. If it's positive on the second occasion, then infection has occurred and she should discuss with her doctor and a gynaecologist whether termination would be advisable. (*See* ABORTION.)

In the UK, all girls aged 11–13 are now offered *immunization* against German measles. Unfortunately, a lot of them dodge the jab! Many hospitals now give newly-delivered first-time mothers anti-German measles vaccine if they're not already immune. But ideally, ALL women should be protected against rubella before they embark on pregnancy.

GIDDINESS (*See* DIZZINESS.)

GLANDULAR FEVER

Also known as infectious mononucleosis, this is a common feverish illness which is almost certainly caused by a virus. It is most frequently seen in young adults, particularly those living in hostels, nurses' homes and similar institutions. The virus is probably passed from person to person in the tiny droplets which are expelled from the mouth when we laugh, cough, sneeze, or even talk. Kissing is also said to play a major part in the transmission.

The main features of glandular fever are usually a moderately raised temperature together with a feeling of lassitude, a sore throat, and enlargement of the lymph glands—particularly those of the neck. There's often a rash at some time.

The illness is often trivial, but may persist for many weeks and be quite exhausting for the victim. Serious complications are rare, and the only real risk is rupture of the spleen, an organ which becomes enlarged with the lymph glands. This disaster may occur if the patient is unwise enough to go in for violent physical activity. In one tragic case, a child died of rupture of the spleen because his mother spanked him during an attack of mononucleosis.

The diagnosis depends on two different types of blood test. These are normally carried out in all suspected cases,

since without them the condition is often easy to confuse with other disorders, such as German measles. There is no specific treatment apart from rest. Avoid a commonly-prescribed antibiotic called Penbritin (ampicillin), which is now known to cause an intensely irritant rash in people who are in the early stages of glandular fever. In severe cases, prolonged convalescence may be necessary.

GLAUCOMA

This is a state of increased pressure within the eyeball. It's not a disease in itself but a symptom of various conditions, in some of which the outlook is more serious than in others.

Acute glaucoma is characterized by quite sudden pain in the eye. The pain is often so severe that the patient vomits. The eye appears red and inflamed, and is often as hard as a golf ball to the touch. Urgent treatment by an eye surgeon is necessary.

In other cases, the chief symptoms are intermittent attacks of dimness of vision with a sensation of haloes round lights. Such attacks often come on in the dark, or when watching TV. Early treatment is essential.

Chronic glaucoma is a rather different problem, since there may be no symptoms at all until the condition is far advanced. Some patients do, however, notice that, as middle age advances, their near vision suddenly deteriorates very rapidly—this symptom should be investigated as soon as possible, though it may just turn out to be due to the normal middle-aged need for reading glasses.

Loss of *peripheral* vision (so that you seem to be looking down a tunnel) is also a possible danger sign.

Ideally, all middle-aged and elderly people should have a regular eye examination every year or so. Indeed, everyone is entitled to one NHS eye check-up a year. If this were done, a good deal of blindness could probably be prevented. The cost of such a scheme would be considerable, however.

GOITRE

A goitre is a swelling of the thyroid gland, which is situated in the front of the neck.

Very slight fullness of the thyroid is quite common in women at certain times of life—at pregnancy, puberty, and sometimes at the menstrual periods. Any other enlargement of the thyroid should be assessed by a doctor, since treatment may be necessary. (*See* **Goitre** under THYROID GLAND in A–Z of Parts of the Body.)

GONORRHOEA

This is a very common type of VD. (*See* VENEREAL DISEASES.)

Its incidence has risen very fast indeed, though in the UK, it has actually levelled off a bit lately—which is not the case in most countries. Two worrying aspects of the disease are *(i)* that in women it may often produce no symptoms at all in the early stages, and *(ii)* that it is becoming increasingly difficult to cure as the germs responsible develop resistance to penicillin. Other drugs are, however, available.

Gonorrhoea, like other types of VD, is to all intents and purposes only acquired by having sex with an infected person. (This need not amount to actual intercourse—other forms of sexual contact can also pass the disease on. This is why, contrary to widespread belief, homosexuals are far from immune to infection.)

A few days after exposure, the male patient often develops burning pain on passing urine, together with a pus-like discharge. In women, there *may* be similar urinary symptoms and possibly a vaginal discharge. Very often, however, the disease remains 'hidden'. Women particularly may carry the germs for months without being aware that anything is wrong, and in medical practice it is common to see girls who have unwittingly infected quite a large number of men, many of whom are quite untraceable. Two-thirds of all infected women do not seek medical aid.

The complications of gonorrhoea are *very* serious, though life itself is rarely threatened. Among some young people, there is a tendency to regard the disease as trivial, or 'like a cold'. This is crazy! In countries where gonorrhoea is rampant, a large percentage of the female population develops completely incurable pelvic inflammation, with consequent life-long pain, discharge and ill-health, as well as sterility. Many men suffer from arthritis, blindness, inflammation of the testicles, abscesses of the urinary tract and urinary strictures, which cause a lifetime of pain and distress. Unfortunately, the indications are that, before many years have passed, we may be facing these problems on a similar scale in most Western countries.

Most (though not quite all) cases of gonorrhoea can be cured by prompt treatment with penicillin injections. Anyone who has even the slightest suspicion that he or she might have been exposed to infection should go without delay to the 'Special Clinic' at the nearest large hospital, and should, of course, refrain from sex in the meantime. Further information is given under the heading VENEREAL DISEASES.

GOUT

This is a condition characterized by intermittent and painful joint swelling, particularly at the base of the big toe. Attacks

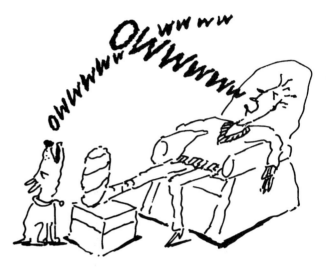

often begin at night; movement is excruciatingly painful, and the affected joint becomes red, warm, swollen and tender. The diagnosis of gout is confirmed by a blood test which measures the level of a chemical called uric acid.

It is an inherited abnormality of uric acid breakdown that is believed to cause gout, which is why the disorder often runs in families. The traditional belief that gout represents the wages of over-enthusiastic pursuit of wine, women and song is mistaken, though it's an engaging idea.

Some people only get one or two attacks in a lifetime, but if gout does keep recurring, then nowadays a wide range of drugs are available to prevent attacks as far as possible. If they do occur, relief can usually be readily obtained with preparations such as phenylbutazone, colchicine, or prednisone.

The doctor will give advice regarding diet and fluid intake, but it is usually best to avoid foods which produce a good deal of uric acid, such as liver, kidney, sweetbreads, meat extracts, anchovy, and sardines. Most patients are advised to drink at least five pints of liquid daily; rich wines are probably best avoided.

GROWING PAINS

It used to be taught that it's normal for your children to feel pains in their limbs as their bones grow, and many people still believe this. In fact, there are no such things as growing pains, and it's possible that some children diagnosed as suffering from this 'complaint' actually had rheumatic fever or some other serious condition. Any child who has persistent bone or joint pain should see a doctor.

GROWTHS

Growths may be benign or malignant. Benign growths such as papillomas of the skin or fibroids of the womb are, of course, relatively harmless, though they may require surgical removal. Malignant growths are discussed under the heading CANCER. Certain common malignant growths are also dealt with under the heading of the organ involved in the A–Z of Parts of the Body (BOWEL, BREAST, etc.).

GUM DISORDERS

These are usually the province of the dental surgeon, and anyone who notices that he has pain, bleeding or ulceration in the gum region should see a dentist right away.

Most gum disorders would never happen at all if people cleaned their teeth properly. This does not apply to gum ulcers and other mouth *ulcers*, however, since these may occur for no known reason. If they persist for more than a few days, dental aid or medical aid should be sought. A number of preparations containing steroids or healing agents such as carbenoxolone are now available, but a few doctors still prefer to treat ulcers with the older remedy of gentian violet, though this does tend to give the mouth a rather odd bright blue appearance.

Bleeding from the gums in babyhood may *very* rarely indicate scurvy (*see* SCURVY).

H

HAEMORRHOIDS (*See* PILES.)

HALLUCINATIONS

In an adult, hallucinations are either associated with drugs, or symptomatic of psychological illness, and the patient must in either case be encouraged to consult a doctor. (*See also* MENTAL ILLNESS.)

In childhood, however, hallucinations are very common with any feverish complaints. If your child starts seeing insects crawling across the ceiling, the first thing to do is to take his temperature. (If you have no thermometer, buy or borrow one rather than ring your doctor to come round and take the child's temperature!) If the reading is high, then it is certainly the fever that is causing the hallucinations. Use the measures outlined under the heading TEMPERATURE to cool the child down.

HALLUX VALGUS

A common deformity of the big toe, usually caused by wearing narrow shoes in early life, and associated with bunions (*see* BUNION).

HAMMER TOE

A toe deformity associated with the wearing of over-tight shoes. Most commonly, it is the second toe which is deformed by pressure so that one of its knuckles rubs constantly against the toecap of the shoe, with resultant corn formation. Surgical treatment may be necessary.

HARE LIP

This is a common congenital deformity. It's often associated with cleft palate (*see* CLEFT PALATE). Although it is a great shock for mother to see her newborn baby's face deformed in this way, she can rest assured that, with modern plastic surgery techniques, it will almost always be possible to put things right. Virtually all such babies nowadays look (and are) completely normal after surgery. Operation is usually postponed until the child is one or two years old, when the parts are larger and easier to work with.

HAY FEVER

An allergic condition, characterized by bouts of sneezing, irritation of the eyes and nose, and copious nasal discharge. The nose runs so freely during attacks that the victim may easily use 20 or more handkerchiefs in a day.

Hay fever is due to allergy to pollen. In some cities. 'pollen counts' are published in the press during the hay fever season. These readings may be of some value to people who can choose whether or not they go out of the house on a particular day.

Perennial rhinitis is a condition whose symptoms are similar to those of hay fever, but which occur all the year round. Here, the allergy is to such agents as animal fur, feathers, or (very commonly) house dust. Recent research shows that the bodies of tiny mites in the dust are the provokers of the allergy, and when this is so it may be practical to desensitize sufferers by giving them injections containing minute amounts of material extracted from mites.

Desensitization by means of pollen extracts is already a possibility in ordinary hay fever, but at present not all that many patients have this procedure carried out. Most hay fever sufferers rely on taking antihistamine drugs but these have the great disadvantage of causing drowsiness. This raises problems where driving a car or operating machinery are concerned; nor should anyone on these drugs take alcohol.

In 1971, a British pharmaceutical company introduced Rynacrom (cromoglycate), an entirely new form of treatment free of the troublesome side effects of the antihistamines. This is a powder which is inhaled into the patient's nose several times a day. It is basically the same thing as the anti-asthma drug Intal (*see* ASTHMA), and has since given good results.

Nasal steroid inhalers such as Beconase are also building up an excellent record. And in 1982, the first antihistamine which does not sedate the brain became available.

HEADACHE

Many people tend to think that a headache is a symptom of some severe illness, but this is very rarely so. Particularly common is the worried person who is convinced that the tight feeling across his forehead is due to a brain tumour or high blood pressure. Quite often such patients have a relative who died of one or other of these conditions and their anxiety, though misplaced, is quite understandable.

In practice, for every headache due to a brain tumour there are literally thousands which are due to worry or 'nerves'. A very substantial number of headaches are caused by eyestrain, migraine (*see* MIGRAINE), and sinusitis (*see* SINUSITIS). Headache is common in flu and other virus illnesses. Among the few serious causes of the symptom is meningitis (*see* MENINGITIS).

Degenerative joint disease (*arthritis*) of the top-most part of the spine (common in the elderly) may cause headache, usually around the back part of the skull.

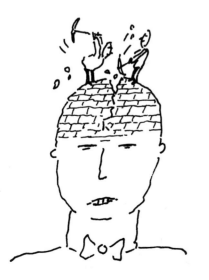

The theory put forward in TV commercials that 'many headaches start in the muscles of the neck' does not cut much ice in medical circles. Nor does the surprisingly widespread popular myth that constipation is a common cause.

If you have a headache, take a couple of aspirin (or some other mild pain-killer) and, if possible, go for a walk in the fresh air, trying to put aside any problems that may have been on your mind.

If you have recurrent headaches, don't brood about them but go and see your doctor and describe your symptoms. He will examine you and, if necessary, order tests to exclude serious disease. But don't delay in seeing him — in all tension headaches, the longer the person waits and worries, the worse the symptoms get.

HEART ATTACKS (*See* CORONARY THROMBOSIS.)

HEART FAILURE

People are sometimes alarmed by hearing their doctors say they have 'heart failure' or 'cardiac failure', terms which they tend to associate with the thriller writer's idea of heart failure: *i.e.* sudden death. In fact, there are many millions of people throughout the world who suffer from heart failure, and some of them have had this condition for 20 or 30 years. The term 'heart failure' simply means inability of the heart to cope with the normal work load of pumping the blood round the circulatory system.

The exact symptoms of heart failure depend on a number of factors, but they may include puffiness of the ankles, swelling of the abdomen, breathlessness on exertion, and inability to breathe properly while lying flat.

Failure may be caused by all sorts of heart disorders (*see* HEART TROUBLE), but most cases respond very well to treatment with drugs such as digoxin (or digitalis) and the diuretics — preparations which help the body get rid of excess water 'left behind' by the sluggish circulation. Other measures, such as a salt-free diet, may also be necessary.

HEART TROUBLE

If you think you have heart trouble, go to your doctor, tell him about it, and let him examine you.

There are a vast number of people (particularly young adults and middle-aged men) who are convinced that they have a heart condition, but who in reality have nothing of the sort. Usually, they complain of palpitations, feelings of faintness, tiredness or stabbing pain occurring below the left nipple. Such symptoms commonly have their basis in stress and strain — the heart being a natural focus for a worried person's anxieties.

These sort of symptoms usually clear up completely when a person has told his doctor of his worries, had a check-up, and if necessary some tests, and been reassured that his heart is sound.

Real Heart Disease

This is not intended to be a textbook of medicine, so there is no need for us to go very deeply into the causes and complications of the various types of heart disease.

CORONARY HEART DISEASE. Ischaemic or coronary heart disease is the commonest type encountered in Western countries. This is the kind of heart disorder often characterized by angina and sometimes the occurrence of 'coronary thrombosis'—or of heart failure. (*See* ANGINA, CORONARY THROMBOSIS, AND HEART FAILURE.)

RHEUMATIC HEART DISEASE. This is caused by rheumatic fever (*see* RHEUMATIC FEVER) in early life, and is now far less common than it used to be. Rheumatic fever damages the heart valves and this may lead to heart failure (*see* HEART FAILURE). Damaged valves can nowadays often be surgically repaired or replaced.

CONGENITAL HEART DISEASE. This is present from birth and is characterized by various types of structural abnormalities of the heart. Until recent years, the death rate in childhood was very high, but modern surgical techniques have transformed the outlook. A high proportion of 'blue babies' and other children with congenital heart disease now do very well.

CARDIOMYOPATHIES. These constitute a special group of heart disorders and very little was known about them till recent years. Their cause is still unknown. Some cases can be treated surgically, but most patients are given digoxin or other drugs as needed. Careful life-long supervision by a cardiologist is essential.

HEARTBURN

Burning pain felt behind the lower end of the breast-bone. Many people experience this symptom at some time (particularly during pregnancy), as a manifestation of mild indigestion. A simple alkali or a glass of milk should provide relief.

Persistent heartburn over a period of weeks may be an indication of the presence of hiatus hernia (*see* HIATUS HERNIA) or occasionally some other condition, and a doctor's advice should be sought.

HERNIA (*See* RUPTURE.)

HEROIN ADDICTION

Heroin is a 'hard' drug, and one of the opiate group, like morphine, methadone, and opium itself. Unhappily, misinformed people still tend to confuse heroin with cannabis, or 'pot' (*see* CANNABIS), but this is a very dangerous mistake. Heroin and other opiate drugs are killers—and they kill fast. The average age of addicts who died in a recent year was 24.

Nicknames for heroin include H, horse, harry, jack, kick, junk, smack, and dope, but new terms seem to be coined practically every month. Anyone who hears his child using these terms should be aware that there is a real risk that the boy or girl may be experimenting with heroin.

To many parents, the very idea may seem ludicrous. In fact, abuse of opiate drugs amongst young people in most Western countries has increased alarmingly during recent years, and literally hundreds of parents have been astounded to find that 12- or 14-year-old sons or daughters have acquired heroin in schools, clubs, or coffee bars. Nowadays, there are few large towns where a teenager could not be offered heroin in a coffee bar (usually, of course, by some 'friendly' person who will assure the victim that the stuff would do him no harm).

Heroin can be taken by mouth or by sniffing, but users generally prefer injection, either through the skin or directly into a vein ('mainlining'). The injection is almost always made with unsterile water, with the result that the user soon develops abscesses and ugly scars on the arms. (Similar infected abscesses in the liver and other internal organs are a common cause of death.)

Apart from scars, abscesses, bruises and blood spots, other symptoms which may alert a parent to heroin addiction include pin-point pupils and a state of drowsy contentment which is replaced every few hours by irritability and anxiousness as the time for the next 'fix' approaches. Interest in work, food and even sex declines, and the young person soon becomes increasingly wasted, untidy and apathetic. As his craving for heroin grows, he needs more and more money to buy supplies of the drug, and he will beg, borrow or steal to get the cash.

Treatment

He is now on a rapid downhill course, and without treatment will probably soon be dead. Even with treatment, the outlook is very doubtful, but some addicts do recover with skilled help, and manage to salvage their lives.

Urgent psychiatric therapy is necessary for anyone who is 'hooked' on heroin. Acupuncture is, surprisingly enough, sometimes helpful.

Nowadays, every parent should bear in mind that his or her child could fall victim to this terrible disease, and look out for the signs. If in doubt, talk to the family doctor (who will *not*, of course, inform the police if the young person does turn out to have taken heroin, though he's now obliged by law to notify the Home Office).

Parents should warn their children from the age of, say, eight to 10 of the appalling risks of experimenting with heroin and the other opiates. Most young people assume that only 'weak characters' can get hooked, and that it would be quite safe to try hard drugs just once or twice, 'for kicks'. Unfortunately, *anyone* can get hooked—newborn babies whose mothers took heroin in pregnancy have actually been born as addicts, while men of considerable will-power have become addicted just because they were given opiates in hospital for the relief of pain.

With heroin, morphine, and any other opiate drug, the only safe rule is—don't start. That way, it's impossible to get hooked.

HIATUS HERNIA

This is a very common condition indeed among middle-aged and elderly people, especially those who are overweight. It has nothing to do with the 'ordinary' type of hernia, or groin rupture.

Hiatus hernia is a condition in which the top part of the stomach slips up through a gap in the diaphragm and into the chest. The main symptoms are upper abdominal pain and/or heartburn. Lying down or bending over may make the pain worse. Belching of air and feelings of distension are common. If bleeding occurs within the stomach, there may be black motions or sometimes vomiting of blood.

The diagnosis is made by means of a barium meal X-ray. Many cases respond to weight-reduction and the administration of antacids, but some patients require a surgical operation, which is usually curative.

HICCUP

There are no miracle cures for the ordinary bout of hiccups (a spasmodic contraction of the diaphragm, which is often, though not always, caused by overindulgence in food or drink). The traditional remedies of breathing into a paper bag or drinking out of the wrong side of a glass may work, but their effectiveness probably depends to some extent on suggestion. Swallowing a spoonful of sugar is said to help some people.

Very occasionally, hiccups may go on for hours on end, and be very distressing indeed. Such cases may be due to some internal disorder, and should be treated by a doctor. Until recently, the record for the longest-known attack of hiccups was held by an Irish-American barman called Jack

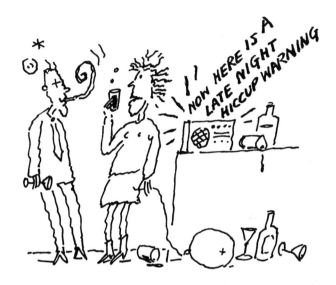

O'Leary who 'hicked' about 160 million times over eight years—and who attributed his recovery to a prayer to St Jude. However, the estimable *Guinness Book of Records* (published by Guinness Superlatives Ltd) has now found a man called Charles Osborne, of Iowa, who has been hiccupping continuously since 1922! Although one is inclined to laugh at such a record, it can't be much fun for poor Mr Osborne, who is unable even to keep his false teeth in.

HIGH BLOOD PRESSURE (*See* BLOOD PRESSURE.)

HODGKIN'S DISEASE

A chronic condition of the lymph glands. In the olden days, the outlook to this disorder was very bleak, but with modern methods of treatment things are much better. Many patients with this condition lead perfectly normal lives, and some are completely cured, though only after many years of regular treatment.

HOMOSEXUALITY

First, let's put the record straight. The average 'gay' (male or female) is an ordinary decent human being, not some kind of monster, as too many people still imagine. It's become abundantly clear in recent years that both male and (perhaps to a lesser extent) female homosexuality are very much commoner than people used to think. The cause of 'gayness' is not known, though all sorts of theories have been put forward. Some authorities think that where children are brought up in a normal, well-adjusted family who have an open, frank approach to sex, there is little risk of homosexuality, either male or female. Others disagree!

There may perhaps be a particular danger where the father is weak or absent, or where the mother is dominating, aggressive, or condemnatory in her attitudes towards the child's sexuality. An extreme case would be that of the overbearing mother who tells her son that everything to do with sex, reproduction and girls is 'dirty'. Such a child would be quite likely to grow up with the fear and disgust towards women and their bodies which is evinced by some (but not all) male homosexuals.

Isolated homosexual incidents between boys do not, of course, indicate that a child is going to be a homosexual. It has been shown repeatedly that such episodes are very common indeed up to about the age of 15, particularly in institutions such as boarding schools. In much the same way, adolescent girls may develop 'crushes' on each other or on a teacher. Almost all of these children become completely normally-adjusted adults, and their childhood behaviour is simply an indication of the well-recognized psychological fact that no one is 100% heterosexual, any more than a person is 100% homosexual. In fact, *bi-sexuality* is much commoner than most people imagine.

In such cases, it is best for the parents to make as little fuss as possible in front of the child. As far as can be ascertained, they need have little fear that the episode will turn him into a homosexual.

Treatment

In established homosexuality, treatment is very rarely relevant—mainly because most homosexuals, male and female, simply *do not want to be 'cured', and feel perfectly normal as they are*. Where an individual actually wants treatment (as may be the case when his personality retains a strong heterosexual component), the balance can sometimes be tipped toward normality by intensive psychiatric treatment. However, Gay Libbers claim that the results of this treatment can be harmful to the personality, and they may be right.

All in all, if you're gay, it's probably best to stay that way and get on with the business of enjoying life. Fortunately, the appalling prejudice against gays which has existed for centuries is now beginning to disappear.

HOUSEMAID'S KNEE

This is an inflammation of a sac of fluid just in front of the kneecap. It is caused by spending long periods of time on the knees, and is common in domestic cleaners and miners though not, oddly enough, in clergymen.

The symptoms are pain, swelling and redness of the skin.

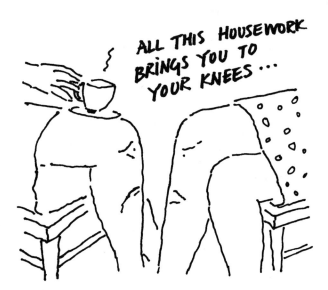

ALL THIS HOUSEWORK BRINGS YOU TO YOUR KNEES...

A doctor should be consulted. He may be able to tap off the fluid with a needle, but an operation to remove the sac may be needed. In the meantime, either stop kneeling altogether or, if this is impossible, use a thick foam rubber kneeler and change the position frequently.

HYDROCEPHALUS

This is 'water on the brain', and is due to a blockage of the channel through which fluid normally drains from the brain. The condition may be suspected if a baby's head seems to be expanding at an unusual rate. Take the child to the doctor for measurement of the skull. If there is any doubt, he will carry out several measurements over a period of weeks.

Some children with hydrocephalus do get better of their own accord. Some others can be helped by means of a special valve which lets the excess fluid drain off from the brain. This valve was invented by an American engineer whose own baby was suffering from hydrocephalus.

While the outlook is undeniably bleak for some children with this condition, others grow up to be healthy adults with normal or above-normal intelligence.

HYPERTENSION (*See* BLOOD PRESSURE.)

HYPERTHYROIDISM (*See* THYROID in the A–Z of the Parts of the Body.)

HYPOTHERMIA

This is a condition of extreme cold, *very* common in old

people in winter. Treatment is by gentle rewarming in hospital. But since hypothermia carries a high death rate, the best thing is *prevention*. Families should take great care to see that their elderly relatives wear plenty of warm clothes, and have plenty of heating, in winter.

HYSTERECTOMY

This is the operation of removal of the womb. It is one of the most common of all surgical procedures, and it is a fair bet that on any crowded bus there will be one or two women whose abdomens bear the small scar of a hysterectomy.

There are many conditions for which the operation is performed, among the commonest being fibroids (*see* FIBROIDS). *No part of the vagina is removed*, except in a very rare form of hysterectomy done for cancer. So the patient's common fear that she is 'no longer a woman', or that she will be unable to continue to enjoy love-making, is quite unjustified. (In fact, many women find sex much more satisfying after hysterectomy, because the fear of unwanted pregnancy is gone forever.) However, intercourse should usually be deferred until about six weeks after the operation, to avoid the risk of disturbing the stitches; the gynaecologist will advise on the exact time when love-making can be resumed.

Removal of the Ovaries

If the ovaries are not removed at the same time as the womb, the woman shouldn't feel all that much physical upset after hysterectomy. Sometimes, however, the surgeon decides that it's necessary to take away the ovaries because they are diseased. When this is done, the woman will often experience some of the more trying symptoms of the menopause (*see* MENOPAUSE). Hot flushes in particular may be very disturbing, but a course of hormones can be given to replace those manufactured by the ovaries.

HYSTERIA

Hysteria is *not* the condition described by certain Victorian novelists, in which people shriek with uncontrollable laughter until they are given a curative slap on the face! ('Thank you, vicar—I needed that.')

It is, in fact, a common form of psychological illness in which the patient (often a young woman—though men are not immune) produces various physical symptoms in which she firmly believes, but whose origin lies in emotional stress. Typically, a girl may develop abdominal pain, paralysis or blindness for which there is no physical cause. She is not, of course, malingering, and exhortations to 'snap out of it' or 'pull yourself together' are not very likely to work.

Mass hysteria occasionally occurs among schoolgirls. In several well-publicized 'epidemics' which have happened over the last few years, literally hundreds of girls who were assembled together kept collapsing and being taken to hospital in droves. Most of them thought either that they had been gassed or that they were victims of a virus. In one case, irate parents threatened a totally innocent ice-cream vendor whose choc-ices they blamed for the problem.

The treatment of hysteria is often difficult. A calm, sensible family doctor can often do a great deal of good by friendly reassurance and the judicious use of tranquillizers over a short period. Similarly, the girl's parents should try not to panic. Nor, of course, should they accuse her of 'faking' the illness. It is best if they simply deal with the symptoms in a cool and collected fashion as they arise. Skilled psychiatric treatment may sometimes be necessary, but people tend to become much less hysterical as they grow up and become more mature emotionally.

I

IMPETIGO

This is a fairly common skin infection, caused by the germ *Staphylococcus aureus*, the organism which causes boils and 'spots', and which is found in many people's noses. The germs enter the skin *via* a tiny crack, often on the cheek or at the corner of the mouth. They then multiply and produce the typical sore impetigo, with its golden crust overlying the inflamed and reddened skin.

Impetigo may spread to other parts of the body which come into contact with the original site of infection, and may readily spread to other people. The first measure of treatment, therefore, is to keep the child away from school. Physical contact with the rest of the family should be cut down as far as is reasonably possible, and the child should have his own face flannel, towel and pillowcase, all of which should be boiled each day.

He should see the doctor within 24 hours of the onset of impetigo, so that therapy with antibiotics can be started. In all but the most severe cases, recovery can be expected within about a week or so.

IMPOTENCE

The American sexual researchers, Masters and Johnson,

claimed impotence to affect 40% of American marriages to some extent, and the same *might* possibly be true of other countries, though figures are lacking. Certainly, the problem is a very widespread one.

Most cases of impotence are thought by doctors to be psychological in origin. Among the exceptions are impotence associated with diabetes and impotence caused by drugs, *e.g.* tablets for high blood pressure, and alcohol.

The majority of patients find difficulty in accepting that their problems are psychological rather than physical, and willingly ascribe their impotence to such improbable causes as hormone or vitamin deficiency, or to advancing age. They may fall into the clutches of quacks, and spend a good deal of money on useless but expensive 'tonics', 'rejuvenatives', and 'aphrodisiacs'. All this is just self-delusion, and, as such, is unlikely to work except by the power of suggestion.

Unfortunately, the impotent patient who goes to his doctor may not always obtain a great deal of help, for several reasons. In the first place, as was grimly remarked recently in a leading medical journal, 'the doctor may be in the same boat himself'. Regrettably, a doctor's training does not usually include any formal teaching on sexual problems, and it is unfortunately true that, in the past, middle-aged men have erroneously been told that their impotence was due to their age. In fact, age is no bar to sexual performance: many men are quite potent at 80 or even 90—and in Elizabethan days, a certain Thomas Parr fathered a child at 105!

Since there is no short and easy answer to the problem of impotence, it follows that effective treatment is extremely difficult to obtain. Patients will often demand hormone tablets or injections from their doctors, before eventually discovering that no magic 'instant remedy' exists.

What can be done about impotence then? At the present time, I'm afraid no wholly satisfactory reply can be given. The first essential, however, is that (after exclusion of the rare physical causes), the patient and his partner should learn to accept the fact that his problem is an understandable emotional one. When this is done, and he recognises that he is not suffering from either some horrible disease or from 'lack of manhood', the problem is then cut down to size, and becomes simply a matter of overcoming his own sexual repressions and anxieties.

A surprising number of men will achieve this victory over a period of time, sometimes aided by tranquillizers or anti-depressants. For others, however, recovery may be very difficult, even with the help of a loving and understanding wife. A 'second honeymoon' together, away from children and the stress of work may be of considerable value.

The most effective therapy available for resistant cases is that carried out at the American Reproductive Biology Research Foundation by Masters and Johnson, but this involves a period of residential treatment for both husband and wife under the care of two highly skilled psychotherapists. It is naturally expensive, and at present is only available to a limited number of patients in the USA alone. The impotent man and his wife may, however, derive very considerable benefit from learning similar techniques to those of Masters and Johnson—and these are taught at some National Marriage Guidance Council centres and Family Planning Clinics.

Good results also appear to be achieved by the treatment known as behaviour therapy—including the form known as *desensitization*, which was principally developed at St Bartholomew's Hospital, London. This is very time-consuming, but an increasing number of psychiatrists, and a few GP's, are learning to use it. For the patient who can afford it, this therapy seems a reasonable choice at the present.

Happily, there is some new research which suggests that in the not-too-distant future, chemical stimulation of some newly-discovered nerves in the area of the penis could provide an answer to impotence.

INDIGESTION

Mild indigestion is very common, particularly after over-indulgence in food or alcohol. Bicarbonate of soda or any proprietary antacid should give some relief. A glass of milk may be helpful. Don't take aspirin-containing pills (this includes most proprietary pain-killers apart from Panadol) as these will irritate the stomach. *See also* ABDOMINAL PAIN.

INFANTILE PARALYSIS (*See* POLIO.)

INFECTIOUS MONONUCLEOSIS (*See* GLANDULAR FEVER.)

INFERTILITY (*See* STERILITY.)

INFLUENZA

Flu is not really one disease but a group of illnesses caused by virus infection. There are three strains of influenza virus (A, B and C) and these produce broadly similar symptoms in an infected human being. These symptoms are fever, shivering, sweating, headache, muscular pains, and feeling generally awful! There may also be a head cold and sore throat.

Such symptoms can also be produced by other common wintertime viruses apart from influenza A, B and C, and in desperation doctors tend to diagnose such cases as being due to flu!

Flu virus A is more common than virus B, and virus C is quite rare. All three can change their nature at the drop of a hat, which is why anti-influenza vaccines are very far from being 100% effective. At present most doctors feel that it is worth vaccinating *people who are at special risk* (bronchitics, etc.) shortly before an epidemic is due to arrive.

But at the moment the Department of Health *doesn't* recommend flu vaccine for everybody—partly because the vaccine can have side-effects.

There is no specific treatment for influenza, though drugs such as aspirin will relieve fever, headache and muscular pains. Antibiotics will *not* affect the virus, but will combat the bacterial infection that so frequently follows within a day or two of the onset of flu. Recent research suggests that new anti-virus compounds are going to prove useful against flu.

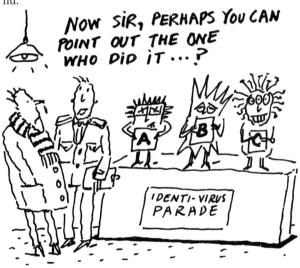

Complications of influenza used to be very serious. Older people may remember that the Spanish flu of 1918–19 killed more people than the Great War did. Most of these victims died of pneumonia, but this complication has been uncommon since the introduction of antibiotics. Post-influenza depression (*see* DEPRESSION) is quite frequently seen, and anyone who does not seem to be 'picking up' and who stills feels weak, exhausted and poorly, three or four weeks after a bout of flu should certainly go and have a chat with the doctor about these symptoms.

INGROWING TOENAIL (*See* TOENAIL, INGROWING.)

INOCULATION (*See* IMMUNIZATION.)

INSECT BITES

These are far more common than people think, and a good many rashes occurring at the wrists and the ankles and under gaps in the clothing are actually due to insects. A common skin condition in babies, called papular urticaria, puzzled doctors for years until it became clear that infants suffering from it were actually being bitten by tiny flying insects as they lay in their prams!

Most insect bites should simply be left alone. If necessary, calamine lotion or a cold compress will give relief from itching. Above all, don't scratch! A high proportion of insect bites that 'go wrong' do so because the patient has scratched them. Proprietary anti-pain sprays Wasp-Eze or PR Spray may help. But pain-killing and antihistamine applications can cause violent skin sensitivity reactions.

If the bite becomes infected or if the surrounding skin becomes grossly inflamed and swollen, see a doctor who will prescribe appropriate treatment, such as antibiotics or antihistamines.

A small number of people seem to be especially attractive to insects and regularly collect an alarming number of bites, particularly when they go into the countryside. Regular use of an insect-repellent aerosol will cope with this problem.

(Bee stings and wasp stings are not, of course, bites and are dealt with under STINGS.)

INSOMNIA

Inability to sleep is very common indeed. Occasional mild sleeplessness when under temporary stress (*e.g.* the night before an exam) is of no great consequence but more persistent insomnia needs medical advice.

For mild sleeplessness, the best thing is to try and put the problems of the day entirely out of your mind. It's often helpful to go through a familiar routine, such as a warm bath, a hot drink and then reading one chapter of a favourite book in bed. Alcohol is also a good sleep-producer, and, particularly in the elderly, a nightcap of sherry or whisky will often work wonders. But for God's sake don't overdo it—far too many people have become alcoholics through using booze as a nightly 'sleeping pill'.

The severer type of insomnia is very often a symptom of depression (*see* DEPRESSION). The person may keep waking up at 3 or 4 a.m. rather than failing to get off to sleep at night. Since lack of sleep in itself is liable to make the depression worse, a vicious circle is set up. Treatment is therefore a matter of some urgency.

If the doctor feels that depression is present, he will probably give antidepressant drugs to be taken during the day. It's possible that he will also prescribe a sleeping pill at night, but not all patients require this. Sleeping pills should only be used as the doctor directs, should not be taken with alcohol, and should be kept in a safe place away from the bed, since drowsy patients sometimes take repeat doses by mistake. Bear in mind that some of these drugs are potential killers, particularly the old-fashioned barbiturates.

INSULIN REACTION (*See under* DIABETES)

INTERCOURSE—DIFFICULTIES IN

Sexual problems are extremely common, and it is quite obvious that the physical side of many marriages is unsatisfactory to one partner or both. The situation does seem to be improving, however, and this is undoubtedly because people in general are today far less ignorant about love-making than they were 20 or even 10 years ago.

Where a husband and wife have difficulties with intercourse, the best thing is if they both sit down and read a good marriage manual, which can be obtained from places like the Family Planning Association (phone number below) or the National Marriage Guidance Council (01-580 1087). Do choose a recent one, however—many of the books which were written a few years back contain all sorts of dangerous myths and misleading information!

A small (but slowly increasing) number of doctors are now undertaking training in the treatment of sexual problems. If your own doctor can't help you, ask him to refer you to someone who can. If in difficulty, ring the Family Planning Information Service at 01-636 7866. (*See also* IMPOTENCE.)

ITCHING

Itching of the skin may be a symptom of various conditions, the most common of which are INSECT BITES (often unnoticed), chemical irritation or ALLERGY (*e.g.* from deodorants or cosmetics), ECZEMA, URTICARIA, obstructive jaundice (*see* JAUNDICE), SUNBURN, and scabies—a disorder which has been on the increase recently, especially among young people. (*See* SCABIES.)

In America, over-use of soap and hot water is, amazingly enough, one of the commonest causes of itchy skin. People who are obsessed with personal cleanliness may easily dry the natural oils out of the skin, and so produce really intense irritation. This syndrome is particularly liable to affect the skin between the legs.

For itching of the vagina and of the anus, see under PRURITUS.

As a general rule, scratching will make any itch worse. Leave the skin alone or, at most, apply calamine lotion. Aspirin by mouth is sometimes helpful. See your doctor if any itch persists for more than a few days.

J

JAUNDICE

Jaundice simply means yellowness of the skin (and the eyes) caused by an increase of a pigment called bilirubin in the bloodstream. It's not a single disease, and there are literally dozens of different causes of jaundice. It is obviously your doctor's business to sort these out and, as this is not a textbook of medicine, we won't go into the complicated details of differentiating one type of jaundice from another. But I'll describe several of the commoner kinds.

Infective Jaundice (Type A Hepatitis)

Infective jaundice (or infectious hepatitis) is the 'ordinary' type of jaundice so often caught by children and young people, particularly in schools, barracks and similar institutions. It is caused by a virus affecting the liver, and is said in most cases to be transmitted by faecal contamination of food or water. The incubation period is usually 28–40 days.

The illness begins with fever, nausea, loss of appetite and a general feeling of ill-health. Smokers often lose all interest in cigarettes. The diagnosis is difficult to make at this stage (unless the patient is known to have been exposed to infection a month or so earlier), but within a few days or so the skin and the whites of the eyes acquire a yellow tinge.

Most patients are jaundiced for only a week or two and then make a complete recovery. There is no specific treatment apart from rest in bed. Some patients are hospitalized, but others remain at home. In uncomplicated cases, special diets are no longer thought necessary. Considerable care must be taken in disposal of the patient's excreta to prevent further spread of the disease, and the family doctor will advise on this point. The patient's family should wash their hands carefully in hot water after any kind of contact with him. Convalescence may have to be prolonged, as the illness takes a lot out of almost any patient. Alcohol should be avoided for six months.

Serum Hepatitis (Type B Hepatitis)

This is an almost identical illness, though sometimes more severe. In this case, however, the virus is often transmitted via injections with inadequately sterilized syringes and needles, or in the course of a blood transfusion. Close personal contact can also spread the virus, and recently it's become clear that gay men are at very considerable risk of the disease, possibly because of their anal contacts. The incubation period is much longer than in 'ordinary' infectious jaundice—usually around four months. Serum hepatitis is very common in drug addicts, mainly because they share syringes.

An anti-hepatitis vaccine has just been developed and is proving highly effective.

Obstructive Jaundice

This is caused by obstruction of the passages which carry bile from the liver down into the intestine, so that bile pigment overflows into the blood. Gall stones are a common cause (*see under* GALL BLADDER in the A–Z of Parts of the Body). Whatever the nature of the obstruction, treatment is likely to be by surgical operation, but some investigation of the bile passages by special X-rays may be necessary first.

Jaundice in the Newborn

Many newborn infants become jaundiced, and if you notice that your baby's eyes and face are acquiring a yellowish tinge, you should contact your doctor. Most cases of jaundice in the newborn are not serious, however, and are simply due to a slightly excessive breakdown of blood pigment. Other causes include Rhesus incompatability (*see* RHESUS FACTOR) and various types of infection.

K

KNEE INJURIES

Severe strains and wrenches of the knee should be treated with caution, since knee disorders can readily lead on to osteoarthritis (DJD) in later life. If in doubt, go to the nearest hospital Accident Department where the doctor will examine the joint and probably X-ray it.

Common results of violent stresses to the knee are torn ligaments, and cartilage trouble. The symptoms of both

conditions are rather similar and treatment of both is by complete rest or by surgical operation at the earliest possible date. (*See* CARTILAGE INJURIES.)

KNOCK KNEE

Mild knock knee (*genu valgum*) is very frequently seen in young children, especially those with flat feet (*see* FLAT FOOT). In very mild cases, no treatment may be required. The orthopaedic specialist may decide, however, to prescribe shoes with slight wedges on the inner side. Splints may also be used in some cases to encourage the legs to grow straight.

A child should be seen by a doctor as soon as his knock knee is first noticed, since in later childhood surgery is usually the only practicable way of correction.

L

LARYNGITIS

This means inflammation of the voice-box, or larynx, which lies within the throat.

Acute Laryngitis

The symptoms are hoarseness, cough, and soreness deep in the throat. Causes include infection (usually spreading either downwards from a cold or sore throat, or else upwards

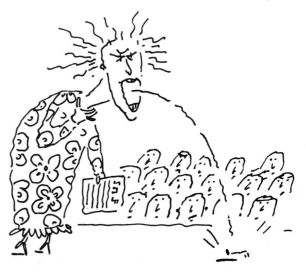

from a chest infection), over-use of the voice, and smoking.

Treatment usually involves resting the voice, stopping smoking, and using soothing gargles. Where infection is present, antibiotics will usually be prescribed by your GP.

Laryngitis can cause croup in babies and young children (*see* CROUP).

Chronic Laryngitis

This occurs mainly in people who use their voice a great deal in their occupations—singers, drill-sergeants, lecturers and so on. Cigarette smoking often plays an important part. The condition may progress so far that nodules may form on the vocal cords within the voice-box. The advice of an ear, nose and throat (ENT) specialist is desirable. If nodules have formed on your cords, he'll remove them.

LEAD POISONING

This used to be a common condition in the days when paints often contained lead, and it still occasionally happens that a child dies as the result of nibbling old paint on his cot. A greater danger nowadays is inhalation of lead in the form of dust or fumes. This is particularly liable to happen among people who work in lead smelting or burning, the manufacture of lead, or the making of accumulators. Also at risk are children who live near lead-using factories, or whose fathers work in this type of industry; lead dust may readily be brought into the home on the father's clothes and hands.

Petrol fumes contain far more lead than is good for the health of our children, and it's time legislation controlled these levels.

The symptoms of lead poisoning vary a lot. They include colicky abdominal pain (still known as 'painter's colic'), anaemia, muscle weakness, nerve paralysis, headache, weight loss, fits, and blueish discolouration of the gums. It seems likely that children who've been exposed to lead actually suffer impairment of their IQs.

Once the diagnosis is made, treatment by means of chemicals which clear lead from the body is fairly straight forward. As the symptoms of the disorder are often rather vague, however, it is all too easy for the patient to die, or at least to suffer neurological damage, before the diagnosis can be made.

Prevention

Lead poisoning can be prevented by careful industrial measures to cut down fumes and dust. People who work with the metal must take great care about getting rid of lead dust from clothes and skin at the end of each shift.

Infants should on no account be allowed to nibble old paint, or to play with such 'toys' as lead accumulators—poisoning has resulted when children have put these on a bonfire and breathed the fumes. And as I've said, it's vital that anti-pollution measures should be introduced and it looks like some measure of control will be brought in by 1985.

LEGIONNAIRES' DISEASE

A dangerous infection caused by a germ (Legionella) which has only recently been discovered. The germ causes a serious form of pneumonia, which can be fatal if the disorder is not recognized. But if the diagnosis is made correctly, the infection can be treated with the antibiotic erythomycin.

The germ appears to have a liking for hot water systems in large 'institutions', such as hotels and hospitals. Unfortunately, a considerable number of cases have occurred in hotels on the holiday coasts of Spain. If one of your family develops an unexplained illness with chest symptoms while on holiday at a hotel in a warm country, consult a doctor promptly.

LESBIANISM

Lesbianism is female homosexuality (*see* HOMO-SEXUALITY.)

LEUKAEMIA

There are a number of different acute and chronic blood disorders which together make up the group known as the leukaemias. Their cause is not known, though radiation undoubtedly plays a part. Survivors of the Hiroshima and Nagasaki atomic bombs had a twentyfold increase in the incidence of leukaemia. Doctors who work with radiation apparatus are considerably more likely to get leukaemia than the average person. The incidence of these disorders is said to have doubled in the post-war years, but whether this is due to additional radiation caused by H-bomb tests is unknown. If so, we should expect some fall off in cases fairly soon as a result of the International Test Ban Treaty, the observance of which has considerably lowered background radiation.

I'm not going to describe the features of the various types of leukaemia—firstly because the symptoms are usually rather vague, and secondly because past experience suggests that some readers would look through the list and quite understandably become frightened that they themselves had leukaemia. In fact, irrational fear of getting this disease is very widespread. Anyone who has this sort of anxiety should see the doctor as soon as possible, since he will readily be able to reassure them.

Treatment

A good many drugs—plus radiation therapy—are now available for the treatment of the various types of leukaemia, and the average life span of patients is now much longer than it used to be. Since the middle 1970s, an increasing number of children appear to have been *cured* of leukaemia —a great advance indeed.

LICE

Infestation by lice still occurs very, very often—even among the most respectable people! The main symptoms are itching and often a slight skin rash. After a few days, it is usually possible to see tiny lice creeping around. There are three separate species of louse, which affect respectively *the body*, *the head* and *the genital region*. In children, it's usually the head that suffers.

Medical treatment within 24 hours is essential, so that further spread to other people will not occur. The treatment consists of application of anti-louse creams or liquids. In the case of head lice (which affect literally hundreds of thousands of kids a year) the whole family should be treated.

Incidentally, head lice are *nothing* to do with dirt, so there's nothing to be ashamed of if your kids get them.

LIGHTNING INJURIES

These are very rare. Essentially they are much the same as electric shocks (*see* ELECTRIC SHOCK in the A–Z of Emergencies). If the patient is not breathing, give the 'kiss

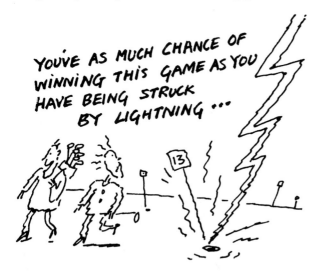

YOU'VE AS MUCH CHANCE OF WINNING THIS GAME AS YOU HAVE BEING STRUCK BY LIGHTNING...

of life'. If there is no pulse or heartbeat give cardiac massage. Both procedures are described in the A–Z of Emergencies, under the heading FIRST AID TECHNIQUES OF RESUSCITATION.

Even if a patient who has been struck by lightning appears to have only trivial injuries, always take him to the nearest hospital Accident Department.

LOCKJAW

Lockjaw, or tetanus, is a very unpleasant and dangerous infection which still causes a number of deaths every year, especially among people living in agricultural areas. Also at particular risk are gardeners, children and sportsmen, but anyone can get lockjaw if the germs which cause the disease chance to enter a cut in the skin.

These germs live mainly in soil (and especially well-manured soil). When they become established in the body of a person who has not had a full course of immunizations against tetanus, they produce a highly dangerous toxin. This chemical causes first muscular spasms (including spasms of the jaws—hence the word 'lockjaw'), and then, in many cases, death. When I worked in an agricultural community in the West Indies, I saw a number of such tragic deaths—they were enough to convince anyone of the need for injections.

Unfortunately, little more than half of all young children are nowadays immunized against lockjaw as they should be. Older children and adults should also maintain full protection for themselves. This is not achieved by 'having had an anti-tetanus jab once when I cut myself', as people often think, but by having a course of three tetanus toxoid injections over a period of six months, with subsequent boosters every five years. Remember that any cut (but particularly any *dirty* cut) may lead to tetanus.

Finally, let's demolish two common myths about the disease. Cuts which cause lockjaw do not have to be between the thumb and forefinger (a common but mistaken belief). Nor does tetanus have anything to do with getting rust in a wound! (*See also* ABRASIONS.)

LUMBAGO

Lumbago is not a disease, as people often think. The word simply means 'pain low down in the back'. (*See* BACKACHE.)

LUMPS

If you find any unexplained lump anywhere in the body always consult your doctor at the next available chance. Delay may be dangerous. (*See* GROWTHS.)

M

MALIGNANCY (*See* CANCER.)

MANDRAX ABUSE

Although it is a useful sleeping pill, this preparation has unfortunately caused a great deal of trouble in several countries during recent years. It became very popular indeed with the drug-taking community, and inevitably many overdoses and some deaths have occurred. Taking Mandrax with alcohol is particularly dangerous. In fact, Mandrax has been officially withdrawn in the UK, but some illegal 'Mandies' are still circulating.

If you suspect someone has taken an overdose of Mandrax, get him to the nearest hospital Accident Department at once.

MASTURBATION

This is a normal part of growing up in many infants, in virtually all teenage boys, and in many girls. People tend to do it rather less with the advent of a stable adult sexual relationship, but as the famous US sex researcher Shere Hite has made so clear, masturbation is a normal part of many adults' sex lives.

Since there are still old books in circulation which perpetuate fantastic Victorian myths about the alleged 'dangers' of masturbation, it is worth stating that the practice is completely harmless. (*See also* PUBERTY AND THE TEENAGE YEARS in the chapter 'The Seven Ages of Man (and Woman)'.)

MEASLES

An infectious disease, caused by a virus which enters the body via the nose and throat. Some parents still regard measles as being a trivial disease, but, in fact, it can have dangerous complications. On the other hand, the majority of children do come through the disorder quite unscathed. The possible complications include pneumonia, ear infection, deafness, eye troubles and, occasionally brain inflammation (*encephalitis*).

As there is no treatment for the measles virus, it is obviously best for children to be immunized against the disease. Measles vaccine should be given to all infants, except where the child's doctor advises against it. In Britain, it's given during the second year of life—but unfortunately many parents don't get their kids 'done'.

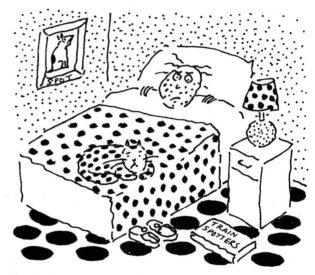

Features

The incubation period is usually about 10–12 days. The child develops a runny nose, watery eyes, a slight temperature, and often a cough. In fact, he seems just to have an unusually severe cold. Inside his mouth, however, there may be tiny little white spots (like little grains of salt) which are the first signs of the measles rash.

The rash itself comes out on about the third or fourth day of the illness. The pinkish-brown spots usually appear first behind the ears, and then spread over the neck, the face, the trunk, and eventually the arms and legs.

The doctor should see the child, but a further visit will probably not be necessary unless there is earache, mental confusion, severe cough or a lot of discharge from the eyes. The child's eyes may be unusually sensitive to the light, and if so his bedroom curtains can be closed. Otherwise, the belief about the light being bad for the child is just an old wives' tale.

Usually, the temperature comes down within a couple of days of the appearance of the rash, and the spots will start to fade shortly afterwards. (Otherwise call your doctor.)

It used to be believed that the patient should be excluded from other children for 14 days after the first appearance of the rash, but many doctors now recommend a much shorter period of quarantine—often seven days where the child seems to have made a good recovery.

MENIÈRE'S DISEASE

A very distressing condition in which there are attacks of vertigo (*see* VERTIGO), together with nausea, deafness, and noises in the ears. Treatment should be in the hands of an ear, nose and throat (ENT) surgeon, and usually involves the use of anti-vertigo drugs. The disorder may go on for many years, but sometimes attacks cease altogether for no known reason.

MENINGITIS

Inflammation of the membranes surrounding the brain and spinal cord, it may be caused by various germs.

Meningitis is commonest in childhood and among young adults. The features include headache, dislike of the light, vomiting, a raised temperature, and stiffness of the neck.

If the doctor has any suspicion of meningitis, he will admit the child to hospital at once. A lumbar puncture will be performed there; this is the procedure in which fluid is tapped off from the base of the spine. Examination of the fluid should enable an exact diagnosis to be made and the correct antibiotic treatment started.

Before the antibiotic era, meningitis killed many children and often left others seriously disabled. Nowadays the incidence of death and serious complications is much lower.

MENOPAUSE

The menopause can be a trying time for many women, but others sail through it without difficulty. A sympathetic and understanding husband and family can do much to alleviate the stresses and strains of the change of life, and an important factor is the attitude of the woman herself. If she goes into the menopause cheerfully, trying to regard it as no more than a minor problem to be got out of the way as soon as possible, she'll probably stand the best chance of an 'easy' menopause.

If a woman does suffer from hot flushes, anxiety and depression, the best thing is to see the family doctor as soon as possible—a sympathetic chat can work wonders, though I admit that not *all* doctors are sympathetic! The doctor can also prescribe hormones and other preparations to help the patient through this difficult time. These can have certain dangers, so women who are having them should have regular check-ups.

Sex life, incidentally, should not be adversely affected by the menopause. In fact, many women find that once they are free of the nuisance of periods and (not long afterwards) free of the risk of unwanted pregnancy, life takes on the quality of a 'second honeymoon'.

Note: If you're having trouble getting hormone replacement therapy (HRT) or regular check-ups, contact the Family Planning Information Service (01-636 7866) who will tell you the address of the nearest Menopause Clinic.

How Should Periods Stop?

Most women are confused about this important point, and a lot of them think that heavy bleeding ('flooding'), or irregular bleeding is normal at this time. *This is a dangerous myth.*

There are only three ways in which the menopause should occur.

(i) periods stop suddenly and never return; or,

(ii) they get less and less in volume until they cease altogether; or,

(iii) they get farther and farther apart in time until they stop completely.

Bleeding between the periods or after intercourse, irregular bleeding, or very heavy bleeding are all abnormal. If you have these symptoms, consult your doctor, who'll probably do an internal examination. He may then send you to a gynaecologist for further tests.

Of course, the cause of the trouble may be something relatively minor, like fibroids or an erosion of the cervix, but only proper investigation will tell whether this is the case. The risk of cancer of the womb and of the cervix is so great at this age that it is essential for you to consult your doctor at the least suspicion of anything being wrong. *(See also* CERVIX and WOMB in the A–Z of Parts of the Body, and FIBROIDS.)

Bleeding after the menopause is also a potentially serious symptom—if it occurs, see your doctor as soon as you can.

MENSTRUATION (*See* PERIOD PROBLEMS.)

MENTAL ILLNESS

The first thing to stress about mental illness is that it is extremely common. It is a fair guess that more than one in ten of the readers of this book will have a major psychogical illness at some time in their lives. A much greater number will have relatively minor illnesses which require only treatment with tranquillizers or antidepressants from a family doctor, as opposed to treatment from a psychiatrist.

This isn't the place to discuss the possible symptoms of the many types of psychological disorder. All I need say is that most minor psychological illnesses are curable these days with skilled treatment (in fact, many such disorders get better *spontaneously* in the course of time). Even major psychological illnesses can very often be cured, and where this is impossible they can almost always be greatly helped.

If a member of your family is showing signs of severe mental strain, then it is absolutely essential to see that he or she consults the family doctor right away. Prompt treatment with modern drugs, combined perhaps with a spell off work and a short holiday away from the cares of the home, will often do wonders for an over-stressed man or woman.

The worst possible thing is for unsympathetic relatives to tell the patient to 'pull yourself together', or 'grin and bear it'. Nowadays, there is no need to 'bear it' alone— effective medical treatment is available, and use must be made of it at the earliest possible moment.

(*See also* ALCOHOL, DEPRESSION, DRUGS—ABUSE AND ADDICTION, HALLUCINATIONS, HYSTERIA, 'NERVES' AND NERVOUSNESS, NEUROSIS, AND PSYCHOSOMATIC DISORDERS.)

METROPATHIA

A fairly common womb disorder, characterized by episodes of heavy vaginal bleeding. Between such bouts, the woman may go for two months or so without a period.

A 'D and C' (dilation and curettage) operation, or scrape of the womb, is often necessary in order to make the diagnosis. Hormone treatment is usually helpful, but hysterectomy (*see* HYSTERECTOMY) is occasionally necessary.

MIGRAINE

Sometimes known as 'sick headache', migraine is a distressing condition characterized by intermittent bouts of severe headache, usually associated with nausea and disturbance of vision, such as 'spots before the eyes'. The pain is often confined to one side of the head, and usually lasts for some hours. The victim dislikes the light, and prefers to lie down in a darkened room. A short sleep will sometimes help to relieve the attack.

The pain of migraine is due to contraction and expansion of large arteries within the skull, but why this should happen is not known. There is often a family tendency to the disorder, and attacks may sometimes be precipitated by eating chocolate or oranges. Psychological factors also play a part —migraine attacks often come on after a period of intense mental work. People who are very conscientious and who tend to worry too much about their jobs may get migraine at the end of the working day or at weekends. The Pill may cause migraine too.

Treatment

It's very important for the patient to relax and avoid emotional conflicts and obsessional preoccupation with work problems. Once he or she learns to adjust his or her way of life a little, the incidence of attacks may drop off sharply.

For the attack, itself, the best thing is rest (preferably sleep) in a darkened room. Ordinary aspirin or codeine tablets are helpful for many patients, but others may need ergotamine—a powerful anti-migraine drug. Because the tablets are often vomited up, an anti-sickness preparation may be helpful. *Very important*: you must not overdo ergotamine-containing preparations, as overdose can actually CAUSE headaches.

There is a tendency for migraine to get better in later life, and some lucky patients who have had severe attacks in their teens or twenties may eventually lose the disease altogether.

MISCARRIAGE

Spontaneous miscarriages occur in many pregnancies. Most cases occur during the first 12 weeks. The symptoms of a miscarriage are rather like those of labour, except that there is vaginal bleeding, followed by painful contractions of the womb. These pains go on until the foetus is expelled. Hospitalization is necessary, and the patient may well have to have the womb scraped (a D and C operation) after the miscarriage.

Obviously, a miscarriage is upsetting, but the fact is that roughly one in every six pregnancies ends in this way.

'Threatened' Miscarriage

'Threatened' miscarriage (or threatened abortion) is the name given to the common condition in which an expectant mother in early pregnancy passes a little blood and perhaps experiences a little pain, *but without losing the child*. If the doctor is satisfied that the pregnancy is still intact, he'll put the patient on complete rest in bed, often under sedation. She shouldn't get up until three days after all bleeding has ceased.

Mothers who bleed in early pregnancy often feel that it would be better to lose the baby, since they fear that it will probably be born deformed. This isn't true, so you shouldn't succumb to the common temptation to try and *make* yourself miscarry.

Warning

In any case of vaginal bleeding during pregnancy, put the patient straight to bed and keep her lying flat. Call the doctor at once. If you cannot contact him, and if the bleeding is heavy or the mother is badly shocked, ring for an ambulance right away.

MORPHINE ADDICTION

Morphine is a highly dangerous 'hard' drug of the opiate group. Its effects and dangers are broadly similar to those of heroin (*see* HEROIN).

MULTIPLE SCLEROSIS

Also known as 'MS' or 'disseminated sclerosis' ('DS'), this is a common and disabling disease of the nervous system, affecting about one in 2,000 of the population of most Western countries. The cause is unknown, but the *mechanism* which causes the symptoms of the disease is a degeneration of the sheath which normally surrounds nerve tissue. There is no reliable evidence to suggest that vulnerability to the disease is genetic, though slightly more women are affected than men.

The symptoms of MS vary wildly from person to person, and diagnosis may be very difficult. (There is, unfortunately, no actual diagnostic test.) People with some medical knowledge sometimes mistakenly diagnose it in themselves.

Among the commoner symptoms are unexplained weakness of an arm or leg, double vision, inco-ordination, and temporary blindness in one eye. Typically, such symptoms clear up after a while—but may then recur after many months, and then go away again for a while.

It can't be denied that in some patients with MS, the outlook is very poor indeed, with eventual confinement to a wheelchair or a bed because of progressive paralysis. But it's now clear that a very high percentage of people with multiple sclerosis do remain well, active and mobile for 20 years or more, suffering only occasional bouts of trouble.

Regrettably, MS is not yet curable—though a cure *may* be discovered in the next 10 or 20 years, because much research is being done on the disease.

But at present, the aim of treatment is to alleviate the symptoms and try to help the patient enjoy as active and mobile a life as is possible. Steroid (*i.e.* cortisone-like) drugs are believed to be helpful in speeding recovery from attacks of MS. In severe cases, good physiotherapy is very important.

Some MS patients suffer from painful muscle spasms, and these can be helped by electrical stimulation or injections round the spine.

Where mobility has been seriously impaired, walking tripods or frames may help the person to get about, often on a temporary basis until the current attack clears up.

I'm afraid that there is as yet no evidence that special diets or added vitamins will help cure MS. But there's no harm in trying any diet (as long as the patient's doctor says that it gives adequate nutrition).

For relatives, the most important thing to do is keep up the person's morale—and to stress to her or him that
(*a*) there are probably many years of active life ahead;
(*b*) a cure could be found at any time.

The Multiple Sclerosis Society headquarters is at 286 Munster Road, London SW6 6AP; tel: 01-381 4022.

MUMPS

A common virus infection. The characteristic feature is painful swelling of the salivary glands, and particularly of the two parotid glands, which lie just in front of the ears.

The incubation period is usually about three weeks. To begin with, the child or adult becomes generally off-colour, loses his appetite, and develops a temperature. His jaws become stiff, so that he has some difficulty in opening his mouth wide. Eating is painful, and the typical swelling of both sides of the face soon becomes apparent. (In some cases, the swelling may be on one side only.) There is no skin rash, and in most cases the patient gets better within a matter of a week or so.

Complications are rarely serious. The virus can spread to other glands in the body (*e.g.* the pancreas, the ovaries, the breasts, or the testicles) but is unlikely to do more than cause temporary pain and discomfort.

In adult or adolescent males, inflammation of the testicles (*orchitis*) *can* be extremely unpleasant for a week or so, and the doctor may decide to give steroid drugs to lessen the

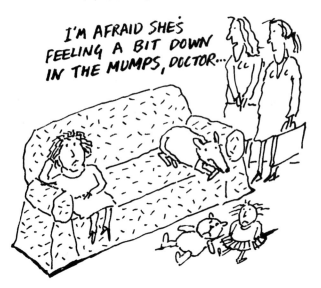

I'M AFRAID SHE'S FEELING A BIT DOWN IN THE MUMPS, DOCTOR...

inflammation. However, the widespread fear that mumps can cause sterility in this way has got a bit exaggerated! It's rare for fertility or sexual function to be affected in any way.

Treatment

Since mumps is caused by a virus—and viruses aren't affected by antibiotics—there is no specific treatment. The patient should rest in bed for the first two or three days. Aspirin (preferably dissolved in milk or some other drink) will relieve pain, discomfort and fever. The patient usually finds it soothing to have a wrapped-up hot water bottle placed over his swollen glands from time to time.

Cold drinks may be appreciated, and a child will often find it easiest to suck these through a straw, since opening the mouth is so difficult. Because chewing is painful, it's unwise to try to persuade him to eat solid food if he doesn't want to do so. There is no point whatever in the old-fashioned 'remedy' of tying a cloth round the child's face.

Usually, the doctor will only need to see the patient once, but check with him about going back to school. Nowadays, most doctors recommend a quarantine of only about a fortnight from the onset of symptoms. Do contact your doctor again, however, if the patient develops pain in the abdomen, the testicles or any other part of the body, or if he becomes confused and complains of headaches.

Vaccine: there is a vaccine against mumps, but it's not given routinely in the UK—except if there's a severe outbreak in a school, student hostel or other institution.

MUSHROOM POISONING (*See* TOADSTOOL POISONING.)

MYXOEDEMA (*See* THYROID in the A–Z of Parts of the Body.)

N

NAIL DISORDERS (For ingrowing toenail, *see* TOENAIL, INGROWING.)

Bruises of the Nail
These are unsightly but usually absorb within a matter of months. If they're painful, however, it's best to seek medical advice. Sometimes it's necessary for the doctor to make a hole in the nail to relieve the pressure—this is quite painless.

Whitlow, 'Run-around', or Paronychia
This is an infection of the nail fold. It often starts in the skin just to one side of the nail, and then runs around to the area near the base of the nail. Symptoms are pain, redness, and swelling. See a doctor, who will either prescribe antibiotics or lance the finger to get out the pus.

Hangnails
These are mainly seen in people whose work involves getting the finger wet—particularly housewives, cooks, domestic cleaners and so on. You need to make an effort to cut down on exposure to water, soap, and detergents, which remove the natural oils from the skin and the nail folds. Rubber gloves should be used, and protective creams rubbed into the nail folds may be helpful.

White Marks on the Nail
These are popularly said to be an indication of lack of calcium, but this isn't so. Most doctors believe these marks are of no significance.

Skin Conditions
These may often affect the nails. They include RINGWORM and other fungus infections, PSORIASIS, and ECZEMA. Treatment may be difficult, so it's essential that it is begun early. If your nails become pitted, distorted or thickened, see your doctor as soon as you can.

NAPPY RASH
Nappy rash affects most babies at some time or other. Its occurrence does *not* mean negligence on the part of mothers, doctors, nurses or anyone else! Some mothers get in a terrible state about their babies' bottoms and exhibit extreme guilt (or extreme hostility) if the slightest trace of rash is present. There really is no need for all this—the rash seldom troubles the baby anything like as much as it troubles the mother, and it can always be cured, given time.

The rash is mainly caused by ammonia, which is formed in the wet nappy by the action of bacteria on the urine. The best way to get rid of these bacteria (and thus stop the production of ammonia) is to boil all nappies, to use antiseptic in the water when you wash them, and to hang them in the sunshine to dry. (The same hygienic measures may sometimes be necessary for sheets or clothes.) Alternatively, use disposables.

Meanwhile, change the baby as often as you can. The more his skin is in contact with urine-soaked cloth, the worse his rash will get. In severe cases, you may have to let the child go naked from the waist down—obviously this means a lot of clearing up after him, but it will do wonders for his bottom! (Nappy rash is not, of course, seen in primitive tribes who don't wear clothes.)

Perhaps most important of all, *do not use plastic pants while the baby has a rash*. These garments prevent the normal process of evaporation from a damp napkin, and thus make things very much worse. Most mothers are so

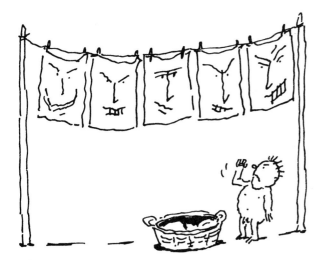

firmly wedded to plastic pants these days that they simply won't believe these facts. Sometimes it takes several weeks before a mother agrees to do without the pants—she's usually then amazed at how soon the rash clears up!

Protective creams and ointments from your doctor do have a place in treatment, but beware of thinking that some magic potion is going to work if you don't use the commonsense measures outlined above.

NAUSEA

The causes of nausea are basically much the same as those of vomiting (*see* VOMITING).

NEPHRITIS (*See* KIDNEYS in the A–Z of Parts of the Body.)

'NERVES' AND NERVOUSNESS

The complaint of 'nerves' has, of course, nothing to do with the actual nerves. People use the word to indicate minor degrees of emotional (*i.e.* mental or psychological) illness, and especially anxiety symptoms. Most such symptoms can be cured or greatly helped nowadays, and anyone who suffers from 'nerves' should not hesitate to go along and have a chat with the family doctor, who can, *if necessary*, prescribe something that will help.

Actual diseases of the nerves (neurological diseases) have nothing whatever to do with nerves or 'being nervy', though patients who have been told that they have 'nerve trouble' are liable to become confused over this point. Neuralgia, for instance (*see* NEURALGIA), is a nerve pain, and has nothing at all to do with 'nerves'.

See also MENTAL ILLNESS.

NEURALGIA

A word applied to any pain arising in a nerve. Common types include the neuralgia which may follow shingles (*see* SHINGLES) and the intensely painful disorder called *tic douloureux*, or trigeminal neuralgia, in which there are recurrent episodes of pain in the face.

Mild neuralgia responds to remedies such as aspirin or paracetamol (*acetaminophen*). Newer and more powerful drugs are available to counteract severe pain. Occasionally, surgery may be necessary to cut through nerve trunks that are producing intractable pain. However, the operation may well leave the affected part of the body completely numb, and this disadvantage has to be balanced against the relief of pain achieved.

There are a number of 'pain clinics' in the UK now, where techniques such as electrical stimulation and acupuncture are used to try to relieve neuralgia.

NEUROSIS

This word just means a psychological illness which does not amount to the severity of a major disorder (or psychosis). Examples include anxiety states and hysterical disorders.

Many neurotic people go through life without ever requesting treatment, and some of them get better of their own accord. It is best, however, to make use of the help offered by the family doctor. He will be able to cope with the majority of patients, but some will need psychotherapy or other forms of psychiatric help. Nowadays, whatever method of treatment is used, most patients can be cured or greatly improved. (*See also* DEPRESSION, HYSTERIA, MENTAL ILLNESS, 'NERVES' AND NERVOUSNESS.)

NIGHTMARES (*See* DREAMS.)

NON-SPECIFIC URETHRITIS

Also known as 'NSU' (a term which is rather confusing in view of the existence of a make of car of the same name), this is rapidly becoming by far the most common type of VD in the UK. Combatting it is likely to be one of the major medical problems of the latter part of this century.

Symptoms are broadly similar to those of gonorrhoea (*see* GONORRHOEA). Prompt and thorough treatment is essential, especially as there are suspicions that the 'bug' involved may cause sterility in women. The disorder is infectious, and patients should refrain entirely from sex until cured. (*See also* VENEREAL DISEASES.)

NOSEBLEEDS

Occasionally (and particularly in older people) nosebleeds may be associated with high blood pressure, and in such circumstances blood loss may be quite heavy.

Most nosebleeds are quite trivial, however, and many children and young people have several such episodes every year. Precipitating factors include blowing the nose too hard, picking it—and, of course, getting bashed on it. Often, no cause for recurrent nosebleeds is apparent. Only very rarely is it necessary for an ear, nose and throat surgeon to carry out a minor operation on the blood vessels inside the nostrils.

First Aid

Sit the patient up, preferably leaning slightly forwards. Tell him that he must breathe through his mouth only for the next few minutes. Then pinch his nostrils very firmly together between finger and thumb, making sure that you squeeze the whole of the soft part of the nose, up as far as the bridge.

Keep the pressure up for at least 10 minutes, resisting the temptation to 'peek'! Then release for a few seconds—if bleeding restarts (which is unlikely) squeeze for a further 10 minutes. It's a good idea also to prevent him from swallowing—you may be able to do this by getting him to hold a cork between his teeth. Continue squeezing until all bleeding stops. Don't let the patient blow his nose, or remove blood clots or poke handkerchiefs inside.

These measures should stop virtually all nosebleeds if properly applied.

OBESITY (*See* FATNESS—no point in mincing words, is there?)

OPIUM ADDICTION

Opium is a 'hard' drug, and its effects are rather similar to those of heroin (*see* HEROIN) and other drugs of the opiate group, such as morphine. Although opium-smoking has sometimes been invested with a rather romantic aura in the past, the reality is that this is a very dangerous drug and no sensible person should be tempted into meddling with it.

OSTEOARTHRITIS (*See under* ARTHRITIS.)

OTOSCLEROSIS

A cause of deafness, especially in the young and middle-aged. It often runs in families, and affects twice as many women as men. Beethoven probably suffered from this complaint. The cause is a hardening of the tiny bones in the middle ear.

Until quite recent years, there was no very effective treatment. Nowadays, however, a number of complex surgical operations have revolutionized the outlook, and hearing can very often be restored to normal or near-normal levels. (*See also* DEAFNESS.)

P

PAIN (*See* ABDOMINAL PAIN, BACKACHE, CHEST PAIN, COLIC, EARACHE, GROWING PAINS, HEADACHE, HEARTBURN, TOOTHACHE.)

PALPITATIONS

People often become very alarmed when they experience palpitations—that is, when they become conscious of their own heart beating.

In fact, palpitations are not often a sign of heart disease but (especially in the young) are more likely to indicate a state of emotional stress. One of the best-known of all the psychosomatic complaints (*see* PSYCHOSOMATIC DISORDERS) is the one known as Da Costa's syndrome, or soldier's heart, in which the patient (usually a youngish person) develops palpitations, pain below the left nipple, and often a fear that the heart is about to stop. Once they've been examined and reassured that their is nothing physically wrong with them, their symptoms usually get better quite rapidly.

In some people, however, palpitations do indicate an abnormality within the heart, but this may not necessarily be serious. If the doctor suspects such a condition, he will arrange an electrocardiogram and chest X-ray, and probably a further examination, this time by a cardiologist.

PARATYPHOID (*See* TYPHOID.)

PARKINSON'S DISEASE

This is the medical name for what people used to call 'the shaking palsy'. It's quite a common illness in older people, and the main features are a curious trembling of the arm, rigidity of the muscles, and lack of co-ordination. There is often an unusual 'hurried' way of walking; the patient takes very small steps and the legs may get out of control so that he has difficulty in stopping. His features often become rather immobile, so that relatives may think that he is not as mentally alert as he used to be, but in fact this is not so.

Some cases of Parkinsonism are due to virus infection in early life; the Spanish flu outbreak of 1918–19 and similar virus epidemics in the 1920s produced a large number of cases of Parkinsonism many years later. In the majority of instances, however, the cause of Parkinson's disease is unknown; although it afflicts men more often than women.

Treatment

The patient should be encouraged to realize that nowadays his case is very far from being hopeless, and that the presence of Parkinsonism does *not* mean that he is becoming senile. Sympathetic help with difficult tasks (*e.g.* doing up buttons) will be greatly appreciated.

A wide range of drugs such as L-dopa have become available in recent years, and most people with Parkinson's disease can be greatly helped by these preparations, though some trial and error may be necessary to find the ideal combination.

Surgery has recently offered new hope for a few patients and especially those under 65. The neurosurgeon carries out a delicate operation on certain nerve centres deep in the brain, and there is often an astonishing and immediate improvement.

PEP PILL MISUSE (*See* AMPHETAMINES.)

PEPTIC ULCERS (*See* ULCERS.)

PERIOD PROBLEMS

The menses, or periods, begin at about the age of 12 on average, though many girls experience the first menstruation as early as 10 or as late as 16. (If the periods start before 10, or if they haven't started by the 17th birthday, it is best to check with the doctor.) Menstruation continues until the change of life (*see* MENOPAUSE), which means that the average woman will have something like 400 periods during the course of her reproductive life.

One still finds patients who think that the female cycle is somehow linked to the calendar (or even to the Moon!), and who therefore expect their periods to arrive on the same day of every calendar month. In fact, the menstrual cycle is usually considerably less than a full month in length—26 days from start to start being about the average. Quite a lot of women have cycles as short as 16 days, or as long as 40 days, and some have periods only once every few months or so.

Irregular and Heavy Periods

It really doesn't matter all that much how long the menstrual cycle is. (There is nothing especially 'right' about a 26-day or 28-day cycle, as a lot of people think.) All that is important is that the periods should be reasonably regular, and that blood loss should not be excessive.

If the periods are irregular, you should always consult a doctor. Nobody need expect their period to come with split-second timing each cycle, but a woman ought to be able to forecast the arrival of her menses to within about two or three days.

Bleeding between the periods or bleeding after intercourse are possible *danger signs* and must not be ignored. See your doctor, who will probably perform an internal examination and, if necessary, refer you to a gynaecologist.

Heavy periods are not only a nuisance but are liable to cause excessive loss of iron, with resultant anaemia. It is largely because women have periods that they're so much more liable to anaemia than men are. (*See also* ANAEMIA.)

It's hard to say what constitutes heavy loss in any individual case, but if you are getting 'flooding' (*i.e.* if ordinary sanitary towels don't seem to be coping with the flow very well), or if regular bleeding goes on for more than six days each month, or if you are getting unusually pale or unusually tired and breathless, then it's definitely best to check with your doctor. He will examine you, and probably do a simple blood test to find out if your body's iron stores have been depleted by excessive menstrual bleeding. If so, it shouldn't be too difficult to put things right. The Pill and similar hormone preparations can, of course, have side-effects—but they are very, very effective in treating heavy, prolonged and irregular periods.

Painful Periods

Pain with periods can be very troublesome indeed. In the past, it was something of a fashion for (male!) doctors to say that much of the distress was purely psychological, and that if the girl would only pull herself together all would be well. This was a rather optimistic view of the problem to say the least.

Period pain is often absent when the menses first start,

but may begin a few months later. The reason for this is that in the early menstrual cycles, there is often no ovulation (see below), and in many patients ovulation seems to be necessary for menstrual pain to occur.

This is why taking the Pill is often a cure for painful periods, since it suppresses ovulation. That provides an effective method of treatment, but in younger girls with only relatively mild period symptoms, it's often best to begin treatment just with simple analgesic drugs. A large number of preparations are now available for the relief of period pain, and the doctor will often try quite a variety before he finds a suitable one. If pain is bad, there should be no hesitation about taking the day off school or work and retiring to bed. A hot water bottle clasped to the tummy will often provide a lot of relief. Anti-inflammatory drugs like Ponstan may be helpful.

Ovulation and Periods
You need to understand the relationship of ovulation (the release of an egg from the ovary) to the menses, since ovulation is the time at which conception occurs.

Most of the time, in most women, ovulation happens a little before the half way point of the menstrual cycle. For a woman whose periods are 26 days apart, therefore, the likeliest time for conception is about 11 to 13 days after the start of a period.

Ovulation varies a lot, however, and there is no way of being *sure*. A slight backache is sometimes a clue to the fact that it is taking place. Some patients take their temperature every morning before getting up and record the results on a chart. A little 'kick' upwards on the graph (preceded by a slight dip) very often occurs on the day of ovulation.

It is also possible to buy 'conception day indicators'. These are just simple calculating devices into which one feeds data concerning the length of recent menstrual cycles. They do make life easier if you have trouble counting off days on a calendar or diary, but as a way of reckoning the conception day they are not as effective as the temperature chart method.

The time at which conception is *least* likely is just before and during the menses. Some people call this time the 'safe period', but this is very misleading; there are hundreds of thousands of children in the world who owe their existence to the fact that their parents believed in the 'safe period'! All that can be said is that it is probably safer than any other time of the cycle'—and the method is certainly a lot better than nothing if your religion forbids you to use other means of contraception. Many Roman Catholic women

swear by the 'Billings' version of the 'safe period', in which you plot the nature of your vaginal secretions on a daily chart.

Incidentally, there is no reason why intercourse should not take place during the menses, where religious prohibitions do not forbid it. A diaphragm or Dutch cap can, if really necessary, be inserted overnight to keep the menstrual flow in check, but should be removed in the morning.

PERNICIOUS ANAEMIA
A type of anaemia (or weakness of the blood) caused by failure of the stomach wall to produce a factor which is necessary for the manufacture of blood cells. Why this failure should happen isn't known.

The disease is commonest in the middle-aged and elderly. The main features are tiredness, breathlessness, paleness of the skin (often with a curious lemon-yellow tinge) and soreness of the tongue.

In the old days 'PA', as it is known, was incurable. (Many of the Victorian ladies who 'went into declines' and died probably had this condition.) In the 1920s, however, Murphy and Minot developed a method of treatment which involved eating very large amounts of raw liver every day. This therapy was effective but none too pleasant. Nowadays, patients are given injections of vitamin B_{12}, usually monthly. The treatment returns the patient to completely normal health, but must be continued for life. (*See also* ANAEMIA.)

PERVERSION
Different people mean entirely different things by this word. It's been shown that where a person hasn't had very much education, he's more likely to regard perfectly normal sexual activity as being 'wrong'. Even today, there are quite a few people around who think that any love-making between husband and wife other than intercourse in the 'standard' position is 'perverted'!

However, most people are rather better-informed than this, and the necessity for various types of love-play between husband and wife is generally recognized. Doctors in the field of sexual medicine do not regard any mutually-satisfying activity which is not harmful as being 'perverted'.

Psychological Illnesses
There are, however, true perversions, some of which are physically dangerous—sadism, masochism, and so on. A characteristic feature of all of these is that the patient only wants satisfaction through his or her deviation and not through intercourse. Quite obviously, these are psychological illnesses which should be treated by a psychiatrist,

if the patient will agree. (If he *won't* agree and you think he's dangerous, then ditch him—fast!)

PETIT MAL (*See under* EPILEPSY.)

PHENACETIN ABUSE
Phenacetin is a useful minor pain-killer of about the same potency as aspirin. For many years, it formed one constituent of many over-the-counter preparations, often in combination with aspirin and caffeine.

By the late 1960s, however, it became evident that overuse of phenacetin could lead to all sorts of unpleasant side-effects, including potentially fatal disease of the kidneys. In fact, the only people at really serious risk were probably the small minority of patients who abuse proprietary pain-killers, taking them every day for years without medical supervision. However, most phenacetin-containing preparations were withdrawn from the UK market at the beginning of the 1970s. You can still find them abroad, however, and they're obviously best avoided.

PHENOBARBITONE—ABUSE AND POISONING
(*See* BARBITURATES—ABUSE AND POISONING.)

PHENYLKETONURIA
An inherited condition, caused by an abnormal gene. Children born with this condition become mentally deficient unless treatment with a special diet is started at the earliest possible moment. The disease cannot be detected at birth except by means of a chemical test on the blood or urine. Screening for phenylketonuria should be carried out on all newborn babies as a matter of routine, and normally is in the UK.

PHLEBITIS
Inflammation of a vein. A superficial phlebitis (*i.e.* of a vein just under the skin) is usually of little importance, but inflammation of the *deep* veins of the leg is often associated with clotting thrombosis (*see* THROMBOSIS) in the vein. Skilled treatment, preferably in hospital, is essential. Usually you have to take anticoagulant drugs to prevent further clotting.

PHLEGM (*See* SPUTUM.)

PILES
It's been estimated that about one person in three suffers from piles (haemorrhoids) at some time during their life. There are two kinds of piles—external and internal.

External piles consist either of skin tags at the margin of the anus or of varicose veins with a thin covering of skin. Internal piles occur slightly higher up, just inside the rectum. They consist of varicose veins with a covering of mucous membrane.

Symptoms
The commonest symptom of piles is bleeding—usually the patient notices a few spots of bright red blood when he has his bowels open. (*Darker* blood suggests bleeding from higher up the intestinal tract.)

Other features include itching, soreness and pain. Prolapse (*i.e.* 'coming down') is a symptom which occurs when internal piles are pushed out during evacuation of the bowels; later, the haemorrhoids may come out spontaneously as the patient is walking around.

Complications of piles may be very troublesome indeed, which is one reason why it is important to get medical advice as soon as you suspect the condition is present. These complications include painful clot formation, strangulated piles, and severe bleeding.

Treatment
Unfortunate consequences can, however, be avoided by prompt treatment. The first thing is to have a rectal examination. This is absolutely essential, because it is *dangerous* to assume that rectal bleeding is necessarily due to piles without exclusion of more serious causes. In the middle-aged and elderly especially, it may be necessary for a surgeon to inspect the lower bowel with an instrument called a sigmoidoscope to make sure no growth is present. Admittedly, in a *young* man or woman, bleeding is very unlikely to be due to anything but piles.

Once the diagnosis is established, either medical or surgical treatment may be employed. Medical treatment is more suitable for mild cases and also when piles are only *temporarily* present as a result of some other condition, such as pregnancy. By medical treatment, I mean the use of soothing ointments and suppositories, plus medicine to soften the stool and make defaecation less painful.

For more severe piles, surgery is needed. Various procedures are available. *Injection* is often used for internal piles, while both internal and external varieties can be treated by the operation of haemorrhoidectomy, which involves tying off the piles and cutting them away. The patient usually has to stay in hospital for a week or so after the operation. New procedures are coming into use which often shorten this time and lessen post-operative discomfort—for instance, Lord's procedure, in which the surgeon stretches the anus (eeek!) under general anaesthesia. For some unknown reason, this helps the piles—and recovery is very quick and relatively pain-free.

PIMPLES

When pimples are really troublesome, the patient almost always has a mild form of acne (*see* ACNE), and medical treatment is necessary. Don't carry on for months trying to treat the spots yourself, but get advice from a doctor as soon as you can, and see him regularly till the condition has gone.

Pimples that occur only occasionally don't need medical treatment. Washing the skin thoroughly helps to keep them away, and exposure to sunshine is also useful. Don't finger them—they're full of germs, and touching them will spread

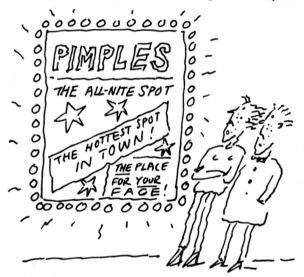

the infection! It's traditional for doctors to tell patients never to squeeze or prick pimples, but this advice isn't much use to the person who is going out on a date and who feels that his or her appearance is being ruined by a large spot on the face.

Under these circumstances, the following first-aid measures are a possibility. Wash the hands carefully with soap and hot water. Then wash the face and clean the area around the spot with cotton wool soaked in antiseptic. Sterilize a pin in the flame of a match and prick the head of the spot. Do not squeeze, as this may spread the infection. Dab the spot with cotton wool until the area is dry. Then apply more antiseptic. Next, throw away the cotton wool and the pin, both of which will be heavily contaminated

with germs. Finally, wash the hands again very carefully.

Failure to observe these precautions may make the skin condition worse or spread germs to other people! (Like to somebody you're kissing.)

PLACENTA PRAEVIA

A condition of the later part of pregnancy, in which the placenta (or afterbirth) lies across the neck of the womb, thereby blocking the way out. This happens in about one pregnancy in 200.

The characteristic feature is painless vaginal bleeding occurring in the last three months of pregnancy. If this happens, go straight to bed and call the doctor. If there is delay in reaching him, it is safer to phone for an ambulance to take you directly to hospital. A Caesarian operation may be necessary, though vaginal delivery is often possible.

PLEURISY (PLEURITIS)

This is inflammation of the membrane which surrounds the lungs and lines the cavity of the chest. It is usually secondary to a lung disorder, such as PNEUMONIA (*see below*). Symptoms vary, but include severe pain in the chest, made worse by coughing or taking a deep breath.

Pleurisy used to be a serious illness in the pre-antibiotic era. Nowadays, it still demands urgent medical treatment and usually, hospitalization, but the outlook is normally very good, and most patients make a quick recovery.

PNEUMOCONIOSIS

A word used to indicate one of a group of lung diseases caused by prolonged exposure to dust. Miners are particularly open to pneumoconiosis. The features include increasing breathlessness and cough, and the production of black sputum.

It's important that the patient is no longer exposed to the type of dust which has caused his condition. Long-term treatment is best undertaken by a chest specialist. The patient should give up smoking and try to avoid damp, foggy air. He should see his doctor whenever he has any kind of respiratory infection, so that early treatment can be given. Industrial compensation is normally payable to patients with pneumoconiosis.

PNEUMONIA

There are various types of pneumonia, but the two common varieties are bronchopneumonia and lobar pneumonia.

Bronchopneumonia

This is a fairly generalized inflammation of the lungs. It's common in the elderly and debilitated, and in the very young. It may follow influenza and other virus infections, or bronchitis. Features include fever, cough and breathlessness. The patient should normally be hospitalized. In strong, fit people the outlook is quite good, but in the very old bronchopneumonia may very often be the final straw which causes death.

Lobar Pneumonia

This is inflammation confined to one limited area (or lobe) of the lung, usually caused by a germ called the pneumococcus. It quite often attacks fit, healthy people, though not as frequently as it used to 30 or 40 years ago.

The onset is usually sudden, with a high temperature, shivering, a hot, flushed face, and rapid breathing. There may be chest pain, made worse by coughing or taking a deep breath. Blisters may develop on the upper lip.

In the bad old days, the patient was usually desperately ill for about a week. At this point, he either succumbed or suddenly began to make a rapid recovery. (This was the moment in romantic novels at which the family physician turned to the relatives and said, 'Thank Heavens, the crisis is past!') Nowadays penicillin or other antibiotics usually start the patient on the road to recovery within 48 hours.

PNEUMOTHORAX ('BURST LUNG')

Spontaneous pneumothorax is quite a common condition in which a lung suddenly collapses. Typically, the patient is a young man who, while taking exercise, suddenly experiences pain in the chest and breathlessness. Some cases occur in Scuba divers returning to the surface, particularly if they have not been properly trained in surfacing drill.

Where possible, the patient should be moved to hospital right away. Most cases recover completely after treatment, which may take several weeks.

POLIO

Polio is a serious infection which is now rare in Britain— but which could make a terrifying come-back because nothing like enough children are being immunized against it.

Poliomyelitis used to be widely known as 'infantile paralysis', but this name is dropping out of use now that it's generally recognized that the disease very often affects adults as well as children.

Polio is caused by a virus which is believed to enter the body either *(a)* by inhalation through the nose and mouth, or *(b)* through contamination of food or water by bowel motions. During a polio outbreak, which *could* still happen

in the UK but which is much likelier overseas, there is a special need to wash the hands after a bowel movement, or before preparing food.

Features

After an incubation period of one or two weeks, the patient begins to feel weak and feverish. His temperature is usually about 101°F (38.3°C). He has a headache with a stiff, painful neck, and he may vomit. If polio is about, then anybody with these symptoms should be put to bed, and the doctor should be contacted. Of course, most such patients will turn out not to have polio at all. If the doctor does suspect polio, however, he will insist on absolute bed-rest for some days.

Some polio patients go through this pre-paralytic stage and then get better. In others, paralysis of one or more limbs develops a few days later. The legs are more frequently involved than the arms. In a small proportion of cases, the breathing muscles are paralyzed and, when this happens, the patient has to go on an iron lung or respirator.

Some degree of recovery of function may be expected with skilled treatment, but unfortunately many paralyzed patients are left with weak and wasted limbs.

Prevention of Polio

Polio could be completely wiped out if enough people were vaccinated against it. It's too late to get immunized when you've caught the disease.

The injectable vaccine invented by Dr Jonas Salk was a wonderful step forward in the prevention of this appalling illness. Nowadays, however, most countries use the Sabin vaccine, which is given by mouth, often on a lump of sugar. Every baby should have a full course of this vaccine with boosters at appropriate intervals. As we've said, adults can be killed or crippled by polio as well. If you're not sure whether you and your family have up-to-date protection, check with your doctor as soon as possible—particularly if you're going abroad.

(See also the sections on IMMUNIZATION in the chapter called 'The Seven Ages of Man (and Woman)'.)

PREGNANCY

The average human pregnancy runs a course of about 280 days (or approximately nine calendar months and one week) as calculated from the first day of the last menstrual period. (Though it's traditional and convenient to count from the last period, the baby is actually in the womb for about two weeks less than the 280 days, since fertilization occurs roughly 12 to 14 days after the start of the menses.)

Pregnancy may be very much shorter than this in cases

of prematurity (*see* PREMATURITY in the A–Z of Emergencies) but the baby is not very likely to survive unless he has been in the womb for at least five and a half months.

At the other extreme, pregnancies rarely last longer than 10 months nowadays. Depending on the circumstances, the obstetrician will usually take steps to bring on labour artificially when the baby is two or three weeks overdue.

For legitimacy purposes, the courts are willing to accept the possibility of a pregnancy going on for about eleven months or so, though some such cases have strained credibility in the past! In the early 1970s, however, it was suggested that some babies could quite genuinely remain in the womb for even longer than this. The theory is that a child may cease growing altogether in early pregnancy for perhaps two or three months, and then restart growth at the normal rate, with delivery occurring after over a year's gestation in some cases.

One such baby born in England in May 1971 is believed by the obstetrician concerned to have spent a total of 381 days in the womb—in other words, a year and 16 days!

Symptoms

The first symptom of pregnancy is usually a missed period. When it's about 13–14 days overdue, it's best to have a urinary pregnancy test done, either through your doctor or arranged with a pregnancy-testing service. Remember, however, that such tests are not 100% accurate by any means; it's always wise to have a medical opinion.

Other symptoms of early pregnancy include fullness of the breasts (often combined with a prickling sensation) and increased frequency of passing urine. Morning sickness (which may, in fact, occur at any time of the day) doesn't usually begin until about the sixth or seventh week of pregnancy.

Antenatal Care

Once you know you are pregnant, put yourself under a doctor's care and make sure you attend the clinic regularly from then on. This really is very important indeed but, even today, one still finds an occasional mother who turns up a week or two before her baby is due, having had no antenatal care at all. Not surprisingly, the incidence of illness and complications in these mums and their babies is very high indeed.

NB There's now some evidence that you should take special care of yourself even *before* pregnancy begins—and

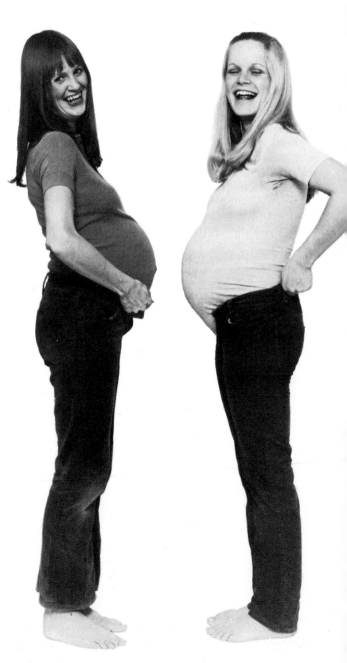

These two ladies may have round tummies—but the rest of them shows that they have kept their weight down admirably.

that adequate vitamin intake before conception will help prevent disorders like spina bifida.

General Health Measures

During pregnancy, try to get as much fresh air and sunshine as you can. A reasonable amount of exercise in the open air each day is a good idea. On the other hand, remember that adequate rest is very important. You need a good eight hours sleep each night, and often a spell of an hour or two each day with your feet up as well. Your doctor will advise on this point.

Don't forget to make sure you have the right sort of clothes during pregnancy. A good supporting bra with wide straps is essential. Note the advice about shoes given below in the section on backache. Avoid tight elastic socks.

Make full use of relaxation classes. If supervised exercises for the stomach and pelvic muscles are available, these are very useful too.

You should only take alcohol in great moderation, if at all, since there's now evidence that it can harm the baby.

Smoking is really best abandoned in pregnancy, but much as I detest the habit—I'd reluctantly concede that one or two cigarettes a day will do little or no harm. Take particular care of your teeth while you are expecting; it's a good idea to get all dental treatment out of the way by the sixth month. If you require an anaesthetic during labour, the presence of badly decayed teeth can make things difficult.

There is no need whatever to avoid having intercourse during pregnancy, unless your doctor advises against it for some specific reason. The 'classical' posture is often uncomfortable in the second half of pregnancy, so it's a good idea to switch to other positions in which the husband's weight is not on the wife's stomach. This can be fun!

Disorders of Pregnancy

ANAEMIA. Every expectant mother should have at least one blood test done, because a pregnant woman has to give a lot of her body's iron stores to the baby—therefore, it's very easy to become anaemic. It also sometimes happens that an expectant mother becomes anaemic because of a deficiency in a chemical called folic acid. Therefore, many obstetricians and GPs give all their patients pills containing both iron and folic acid throughout the pregnancy.

Occasionally, a mother is so anaemic that she has to have a 'top-up' in the form of an iron infusion into a vein, or a blood transfusion. (*See also* ANAEMIA.)

BACKACHE. This is very common in pregnancy, especially where posture is poor. Avoid very high-heeled shoes, which increase the strain on the spine. Advice from the doctor or going to the relaxation class may be helpful. You can try manipulation, but of course you ought to take the precaution of telling the osteopath or doctor that you're pregnant. Rest is essential. A firm supporting maternity corset may be necessary in some cases. Avoid drugs if you can. (*See also* BACKACHE.)

BLEEDING. There are various causes of vaginal bleeding during pregnancy, including miscarriage and placenta praevia (*see* MISCARRIAGE and PLACENTA PRAEVIA). The essential thing to realize is this: if you bleed from the vagina, go straight to bed and phone the doctor. If there is delay in reaching him, and if bleeding is heavy, it's better to call an emergency ambulance to take you straight to hospital. This is particularly true in the last three months of pregnancy when hospitalization is going to be necessary anyway.

ECTOPIC PREGNANCY (See ECTOPIC PREGNANCY.)

MISCARRIAGE (See MISCARRIAGE.)

PRE-ECLAMPSIA (Toxaemia). A very large number of pregnant women (probably about 10%) develop this condition. Fortunately, with modern antenatal care, very few of them go on to the very serious condition called 'eclampsia', which is characterized by severe convulsions, and which may even be fatal.

Pre-eclampsia usually appears after the seventh month of pregnancy. The features are swelling of the ankles and fingers, elevation of the blood pressure, and the passing of protein in the urine. (This is why, at the antenatal clinic, the doctor always checks the blood pressure and tests the urine.)

Pre-eclampsia may have serious consequences for the baby as well as the mother, if it's not treated. It's absolutely essential, therefore, to follow the doctor's advice, particularly as regards rest in bed. Some mothers with toxaemia tend to think that, as they feel perfectly well, rest isn't necessary for them. This is a very dangerous idea, as pre-eclampsia can get worse very suddenly. *A patient who doesn't rest when she is advised to may risk her baby's life and health, and her own.*

URINARY DISORDERS. These are extremely common in pregnancy, and it is important that they should be treated promptly and thoroughly because of the risk of serious complications.

Features of urinary trouble include noticeable frequency and/or pain on passing water, inability to pass more than a very small quantity at a time, and getting up at night to pass water. If you have any of these symptoms (and even if you think it's 'just a mild attack of cystitis') go to your doctor within 24 hours, so that he can send a urine specimen to the lab and start you on treatment, pending the result of the test. (*See also* CYSTITIS, PYELITIS.)

VOMITING IN PREGNANCY. Minor sickness occurring between about the sixth and the sixteenth weeks of pregnancy is very common. Where the vomiting occurs in the morning ('morning sickness'), it's often helpful if the mother-to-be has a cup of tea or coffee or some dry toast or a biscuit before getting up in the morning.

If the vomiting occurs at other times, the patient should try the effect of eating small snacks every two hours or so during the day. It can be a good idea to get someone else to do the cooking for a couple of days, because kitchen smells may provoke nausea. Vitamin B_6 tablets may help.

If these simple measures don't work within a day or two, have no hesitation about consulting your doctor. Prolonged or severe vomiting *(hyperemesis)* can be extremely dangerous to health if not treated promptly. (*See also* ABORTION, BLOOD PRESSURE, HEARTBURN, MISCARRIAGE, PILES, CONTRACEPTION, RHESUS FACTOR, VARICOSE VEINS; LABOUR and PREMATURITY in the A–Z of Emergencies; VAGINA in the A–Z of Parts of the Body.)

PROLAPSE (*See* WOMB in the A–Z of Parts of the Body.)

PRURITUS

Pruritus literally means itching (*see* ITCHING), but the word is usually used to mean itching of either the vaginal opening *(pruritus vulvae)* or of the back passage *(pruritus ani)*.

Vulval and Vaginal Pruritus

Itching of the vulva and vagina is a trying and embarrassing symptom for many women. There are various possible causes. It may be necessary to examine the urine for sugar (which might indicate diabetes). Bacteriological swabs from the vagina should usually be sent to the lab, particularly if there is a discharge present, as is often the case. Frequently, examination of these swabs will reveal the presence of thrush (also known as Monilia or Candida) or of another organism called *Trichomonas vaginalis*, sometimes confusingly known as TV. (*See* THRUSH, and TRICHOMONAS INFECTION OF THE VAGINA.)

Other causes of vulval irritation include ringworm, and other skin conditions, as well as allergy to vaginal deodorants, contraceptive foams, soaps and bubble baths.

Anal Pruritus

Irritation of the back passage is a very widespread problem, especially in men. A lot of doctors think that psychological factors play a part in at least some cases, but they could be wrong! Physical factors include inflamed piles (*see* PILES), and anal eczema (*see* ECZEMA), which is very common indeed and which responds well to steroid ointments.

Threadworms and fungus infections can produce intense pruritus, and the symptoms can also follow the taking of antibiotics by mouth. Over-vigorous wiping of the anal region after defaecation can also lead to irritation, as can too many hot baths.

PSORIASIS

A common and very trying skin disorder, with no known cause. It is not infectious. The characteristic feature is the occurrence of rough, reddened areas of skin on which there are small whitish scales. Any part of the skin may be affected, but the elbows and knees are very often involved. Nail and joint troubles may sometimes accompany the skin disorder.

The treatment of psoriasis used to be much more difficult than it is today. Nowadays, the steroid applications give good results, though some patients respond to the older skin preparations. A few dermatologists give patients ray therapy or drugs to reduce the number of white cells in the blood, but not all authorities agree with these measures.

Sunlight is often very helpful, and there's a special resort on the Dead Sea where people who can afford the trip go to spend a month or so in the unique type of sunlight which is found there.

A fairly new development is 'PUVA' therapy, in which a drug called 'psoralen' is combined with ultra-violet light. Whatever treatment is used, most patients can be greatly helped, though few are completely cured of the disorder. The Psoriasis Society can be contacted on Northampton 711129.

PSYCHIATRIC ILLNESS (*See* MENTAL ILLNESS.)

PSYCHOSOMATIC DISORDERS

It is now widely recognized that the mind has a considerable influence on the body, and on its physiological changes. A lot of people still don't like this idea, and are annoyed by the suggestion that the physical symptoms they experience may have some basis in emotional stress or worry!

But a moment's thought is enough to tell us that when we are excited, angry, or frightened, our hearts pound, our pulses race, and our skins change colour, becoming red or sometimes white. Scientific measurement shows that, under the influence of emotion, many other changes take place inside the body.

It's not surprising, therefore, that stress can easily lead to perfectly genuine physical symptoms such as palpitations, headache, feelings of tightness or of lumps in the throat, and pains in various places. Where such symptoms are largely psychological in origin, the patient will very often get better once the doctor has examined him or her, explained that there is no physical disease present and, if necessary, prescribed therapy to help underlying emotional stress or worry.

In some patients, stress does seem to contribute to actual *physical* disease—the condition of duodenal ulcer is a case in point (*see* Peptic Ulcer under ULCERS). Some years ago it was fashionable to describe a wide range of physical conditions (including 'coronaries', diabetes and strokes) as being 'psychosomatic'. Nowadays, doctors tend to take the view that most of these diseases have multiple and complex causes which we do not fully understand. Certainly, stress may be a factor in some of them, but this is obviously very hard to prove one way or the other. However, research shows that the more stress you've had in the last year, the more likely you are to become physically ill—so be warned!

PULMONARY EMBOLISM

A condition which occurs when a piece of clot (or thrombus) from a vein in the legs or lower part of the body breaks off and is carried to the lungs, where it jams.

Pulmonary embolism is a very common cause of serious illness and even death. It's curious that most members of the public have never even heard of this condition, but it has received far less publicity than, say, coronary thrombosis. This is a pity, because pulmonary embolism is often preventable.

Features

What usually happens is that the patient has been in bed for a few days, often recovering after a surgical operation or childbirth. He or she develops a thrombosis in the deep veins of the leg or the veins of the pelvic region; unfortunately, the clot may produce no symptoms.

A piece of thrombus then breaks off and travels up to the chest, where it blocks one of the branches of the artery that supplies the lungs. Symptoms may include chest pains, collapse, breathlessness, fever, cough, and the production of pink or blood-stained sputum. Skilled hospital treatment from this stage on is obviously essential.

Prevention

People don't realize that, even if you are pretty healthy,

there is a considerable risk of pulmonary embolism occurring if you go to bed for a few days. This is why doctors try to get patients out of bed as soon as possible.

If you have to stay flat on your back, try to spend at least two periods of half an hour each day in exercising your legs. In many hospitals, physiotherapists go round each morning encouraging patients to carry out these exercises at the hospital, and to do them later on, at home.

The Pill can also cause pulmonary embolism, so people with a history of clots in the leg veins shouldn't take it.

PYELITIS (*PYELONEPHRITIS*)

This is inflammation of the kidney, caused by infection with germs. It may be acute or chronic.

Acute Pyelitis

This is caused by germs ascending to the kidneys from the bladder, often after an attack of cystitis (*see* CYSTITIS). It is particularly common during pregnancy. The features include a high temperature, often with uncontrollable shivering (rigors), and pain in the flank and the back, just below the ribs and immediately to the right or left of the spine. Urinary symptoms (frequency of passing water, getting up at night, and pain on urinating) may be prominent.

Acute pyelitis used to be regarded as a trivial condition —'a chill on the kidney'. It's now recognized that this is not the case. Urgent treatment with antibiotics is needed, together with careful lab tests of the urine and in many cases investigation of the whole urinary tract by means of X-rays.

Chronic Pyelitis

Where treatment of acute pyelitis is inadequate or unsuccessful, chronic kidney inflammation can result. This may lead to kidney failure or high blood pressure. It's obvious, therefore, that acute pyelitis, cystitis, or any type of urinary infection must be treated promptly and thoroughly. If you suspect you have any kind of kidney or urinary complaint, see your doctor right away so that he can take action before things go too far. (*See also* KIDNEYS in the A–Z of Parts of the Body, and CYSTITIS.)

PYLORIC STENOSIS

A condition seen in newborn babies (rarely after the second month of life). The child vomits all feeds back with considerable force, and rapidly becomes very ill as a result. The condition is due to a tight knot of muscle at the exit of the stomach. A fairly straightforward operation provides complete cure.

Q

QUARANTINE

In the old days, people used to be very strict about enforcing a 'quarantine' (which originally meant a period of 40 days) when someone had been in contact with an infectious disease.

These days, it's recognized that such strict segregation probably did little good—except in the case of a few very serious and highly-contagious infections like smallpox.

So, for the ordinary childhood illnesses there are now no 'officially recognised' quarantine periods. However, schools, colleges or local authorities are perfectly entitled to insist on their own laid-down periods of quarantine, which vary a lot from place to place. The school or your own doctor will advise you of current local practice.

The only common conditions in which quarantining of contacts may be necessary are German measles (because of its possible effect on pregnant women); whooping cough (because it may be very serious if transmitted to a young baby); mumps (because there's a small risk of giving an adult male a painful case of inflammation of the testicles); and chicken pox (because of the risk of giving shingles to adults—especially the elderly). Be guided by your GP's advice—and, in particular, don't commit the all-too-common folly of taking a child who's been in contact with German measles into anywhere where he could encounter pregnant women. It's amazing how many people are daft enough to bring such a child to a doctor's surgery—which is *just* the place for him to meet an expectant mother.

QUINSY

A swelling in the back of the throat, just by the tonsil. The symptoms are soreness of the throat, intense pain on swallowing, and difficulty in opening the mouth. Quinsy is an extremely unpleasant illness to have, and medical advice should be sought without delay. Meanwhile, use hot salt water gargles and take crushed-up aspirin tablets. Antibiotic therapy should produce relief in a matter of 24–48 hours.

There's a very similar condition in which the uvula—the dangly thing at the back of the throat—gets inflamed and swells up. This is particularly common after a wisdom tooth extraction. As with quinsy, there's pain in the throat and great difficulty in swallowing. Use hot salt water gargles and see a doctor as soon as possible.

R

RABIES

A fatal disease caused by a virus acquired from dogs and other animals. A few countries which practise strict quarantine regulations for incoming animals are free of the disease. These territories include Britain, Ireland, Australia, most West Indian islands and most of the Scandinavian nations.

Anywhere else in the world, you should see a doctor at once if you are bitten by a dog (or any other mammal), so that you can have anti-rabies immunization—which you may have to INSIST on. *Warning*: rabid dogs may appear perfectly healthy in every way for periods of six months or more. (*See also* DOG BITES in the A–Z of Emergencies.)

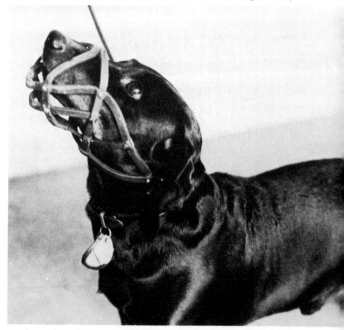

RASHES

Even moderately accurate diagnosis of skin rashes takes years to learn, so I certainly don't propose to try and teach it here! However, it's worthwhile knowing when you should consult a doctor if one of your family has a rash—with or without a temperature.

Some people get very panicky about rashes and summon the doctor at once if they notice a few spots in the middle of the night. This attitude is probably due to half-remembered fears of smallpox outbreaks and other dreadful epidemics. In fact, most rashes are pretty harmless and are often due to some minor allergy. Frequently, they require no treatment and will go away of their own accord within a few hours.

Rashes in Babies

All babies with rashes should be seen by a doctor, though not necessarily immediately.

If a baby has a rash *and a temperature*, phone the doctor, tell him what the thermometer reading is, and ask for advice. If you haven't got a thermometer, buy or borrow one. (For method of taking temperatures, *see* TEMPERATURE.)

If the baby has no temperature, take him along to the doctor the following morning. No treatment may be needed, but it's as well to let the doctor see the child's skin, just in case.

Rashes in Schoolchildren

Take the child's temperature. If it's raised, keep him away from school and ask the doctor to call later the same day.

If the temperature isn't raised, however, and if the child seems completely well, it's likely that the rash is of little significance. If it goes away later the same day, assume it was just a 'nettle rash' and forget about it. If it hasn't gone by the following morning, take the child to the doctor.

Rashes in Teenagers and Adults

Rashes caused by generalized infection (measles, German measles, chicken pox, etc.) are relatively uncommon in these age groups, and most, though not all, eruptions are due to mild allergies or to specific skin disorders (*see* ACNE, ALLERGIES, BARBER'S ITCH, ECZEMA, ERYSIPELAS, IMPETIGO, INSECT BITES, PSORIASIS, RINGWORM, SCABIES and SHINGLES.) In general, if you have a rash that has persisted for 24 hours or more, go and see your doctor.

RECTAL DISORDERS

If you have pain, discomfort or bleeding in the region of the rectum, see your doctor as soon as you can for an internal examination. Don't delay more than a day or two. The trouble may simply be piles (*see* PILES) or some very trivial complaint, but it could also be something serious. Putting off the examination might be dangerous, particularly if you are middle-aged or elderly. Some doctors think that everyone over the age of 45 should have an annual rectal examination.

RETENTION OF URINE

Acute retention occurs mainly in men, and measures for avoiding it are discussed under PROSTATE GLAND in the A–Z of Parts of the Body.

If you find that you cannot empty the bladder, don't make the mistake of drinking more fluid to try and force the urine through—this will only make things worse.

Instead, get into a warm bed and place a hot water bottle over the lower abdomen. After ten minutes of complete relaxation, get up, turn on all the taps in the bathroom, and try to pass water.

If this fails, immerse yourself in a warm bath for 20 minutes or so and then, without getting up, try to empty the bladder into the bathwater.

If these measures don't succeed, call your doctor. He will either pass a catheter up the urinary passage, or (much more commonly these days) send you into hospital for the catheter to be passed.

Prostate surgery (described under PROSTATE GLAND in the A–Z of Parts of the Body) is often considered necessary after a patient has had one or two attacks of retention.

RHESUS FACTOR

In the Rhesus blood grouping system, all human beings are either Rhesus-positive or Rhesus-negative. (In the West, the proportion is about 85% positive to 15% negative.)

Mismatched Blood Transfusion

When a Rhesus-negative person has a blood transfusion, it's important that he or she is not given Rhesus-positive blood. This might cause no obvious trouble the first time, but antibodies against Rhesus-positive blood would be formed in the patient's body. The next time Rhesus-positive blood was given, there would be a violent reaction. In the case of a woman, there might also be trouble with subsequent pregnancies. If the baby were Rhesus-positive, some of his blood cells might leak into the mother's circulation and react with the antibodies which had been formed there.

Rhesus Babies

Today, it doesn't usually occur like that, however, because mismatched blood transfusions are now very rare.

What usually happens is this. A rhesus-negative woman marries a Rhesus-positive man (a situation that occurs in roughly one marriage in eight). If the woman then has a Rhesus-positive baby, some of the infant's blood may leak into the mother's bloodstream; antibodies will be produced in response.

All will go well in this pregnancy, but next time the mother becomes pregnant with a Rhesus-positive child, trouble may result. If her antibodies 'attack' the new baby's blood cells he will probably become anaemic and jaundiced.

Some Rhesus babies are only mildly affected, and get better without any treatment. Others need a complete 'exchange-transfusion' of their blood shortly after birth, to prevent the jaundice from damaging the brain. It is even possible to carry out an exchange of the blood while the child is still in the womb.

Now, most Rhesus-negative mothers married to Rhesus-positive men never have any trouble at all with their babies. But it's fairly easy for obstetricians to be forewarned of possible difficulty by doing blood tests on all Rhesus-negative women, and seeing if antibodies are present in the blood and whether they increase during the pregnancy. Appropriate measures can then be taken to treat the baby.

Prevention of Rhesus Disease

It is now possible to give all Rhesus-negative mothers, from their first pregnancy onwards, an injection of a preparation called Rhesus immunoglobulin. Administered just after delivery, the immunoglobulin neutralizes any of the baby's red blood cells which have leaked into the maternal circulation. This prevents the mother from ever producing antibodies.

This is a great advance, and it looks as though the universal application of this method of prevention will soon virtually wipe out a disease that, until quite recently, claimed the lives of many babies and damaged the brains of countless others.

RHEUMATIC FEVER

A serious condition affecting the joints and other parts of the body, often including the heart. It is fortunately encountered much less often today than it used to be—90% of cases occur between the ages of eight and 15.

The precise cause of rheumatic fever is not known for certain, but in most cases the disease is almost certainly an abnormal reaction to a throat infection caused by a common germ, the streptococcus.

One to three weeks after the original sore throat or bout of tonsillitis, the child develops a temperature and complains of pains in one or more of the large joints (the knees, wrists, ankles and elbows). The joint is usually swollen and stiff.

If your child has these symptoms, put him straight to bed and ask the doctor to call the same day. Quiet and rest are essential from the start if heart valve damage, which is

the most serious complication of rheumatic fever, is to be avoided. (*See* HEART TROUBLE.)

The doctor will probably give a course of penicillin, plus aspirin in quite hefty doses. Steroids (cortisone-like drugs) are also sometimes used.

The child who has recovered from rheumatic fever need not be cossetted and treated like an invalid, but it's very important that for some years thereafter he takes antibiotics as prescribed by the doctor with unfailing regularity. If he develops a sore throat or tonsillitis, he should see the doctor the same day, as a change of antibiotic will probably be necessary. He will also need special antibiotic 'cover' for all future visits to the dentist.

'RHEUMATISM'

There is actually no such condition as rheumatism! This news comes as a surprise to most people, since the idea of such a disorder is so entrenched in popular speech, along with those other 'non-diseases', fibrositis, lumbago, sciatica and so on.

Doctors still occasionally use the term 'acute rheumatism' to refer to rheumatic fever (*see* RHEUMATIC FEVER), but this is not what the public mean by rheumatism.

What a person is implying when he says he 'has rheumatism' is that he regularly gets pain in his joints or, less commonly, his muscles, ligaments and tendons. This pain may be due to a wide variety of causes, but most commonly to degenerative joint disease (DJD) or osteoarthritis, which is fully dealt with under the heading ARTHRITIS.

Anyone who has any kind of 'rheumatic' pain should seek medical advice and not just accept the symptoms as being an inevitable consequence of growing older. Modern methods of precise diagnosis and treatment of musculoskeletal disorders have revolutionized the position for many people for whom life was once a painful burden.

RHEUMATOID ARTHRITIS (RA)

This common disorder is a form of joint inflammation. (*Note*: there are many other forms of arthritis. *See* ARTHRITIS.) Women are affected three times as often as men, and the average age of onset is about 35–40. There is also a children's form of the disease (*see* STILL'S DISEASE).

When rheumatoid arthritis begins, there is often a period of rather vague ill-health lasting a few weeks or sometimes longer. The diagnosis is difficult to make at this stage except with the aid of special tests.

Sooner or later, the patient develops the characteristic features of the disease, which are pain and swelling of the small joints of the hands. Inflammation may also spread to the wrists, elbows and feet, and sometimes to the other limb joints.

Regular treatment under the direction of a specialist in internal medicine or a rheumatologist is desirable. Important measures include adequate rest, splinting of the joints, warmth, and special exercises. Some patients become anaemic, and iron therapy may be needed. Many valuable drugs, including plain aspirin, gold, steroids, and ACTH are now available for the treatment of rheumatoid arthritis.

In recent years, corrective surgery has opened up exciting new prospects for patients whose hands have been deformed by this disorder. Not all patients are suitable for operation, however.

In some sufferers, particularly those who develop the condition late in life, the disease may eventually 'burn itself out'. All in all, the outlook in rheumatoid arthritis is very much better these days than it used to be.

RICKETS

A childhood condition which causes appalling bone deformities. Rickets used to be very common in all the great industrial cities of the world, but it is fortunately rare nowadays. This is because of the fact that in most Western countries today many infants are given vitamin D routinely, often in the form of fish liver oils. This vitamin protects children against rickets. (There is a little vitamin D in butter and eggs, but this may not be enough for a growing child.)

Some doctors argue that rickets is not strictly speaking a vitamin deficiency, but rather a 'sunshine deficiency'. Sunshine manufactures vitamin D in people's skins. A child who lives in the clean, unpolluted air of the countryside, and who spends most of his time out in the open with his skin exposed to the sunshine, stands virtually no chance of ever getting rickets.

In cities, however (and particularly cities far from the Equator), the sunlight has to fight its way through thick layers of cloud, smoke, soot and smog. Obviously, infants can manufacture little vitamin D of their own under such circumstances.

The children of black and Asian people who move to industrial Northern towns and cities are at particular risk, because the sun finds more difficulty in penetrating dark skins than white ones. This is why there have been a number of cases of rickets in children of Asians living in Glasgow and Manchester in recent years. Encouraging these children to get out in the open—and perhaps adding vitamin D to chapati flour—should help wipe out this problem.

RINGWORM

An infection of the scalp or other area of skin by a fungus. (Despite the name, ringworm is nothing to do with worms.)

The infection may be caught from a pet or other animal, or from another person. Because the condition is moderately contagious, it's best to keep close physical contact with other people to a minimum until the patient is cured.

Ringworm characteristically produces small red, rough patches on the skin. These are circular in shape, and the edge of each ring is slightly bumpy. The circles tend to increase in size as the days go by. On the scalp, the patches are scaly-looking, and the hairs in the affected area break off, so that the patient may have quite an extensive bald patch.

Modern drugs available for the treatment of ringworm will usually clear it up fairly quickly, but it's important to see the doctor as soon as possible before the infection gets more deeply entrenched or spreads to other people. The doctor may just prescribe an anti-fungal cream—but if the infection is deep-seated or in the nails, it can now be cured with a long course of a drug called *griseofulvin*.

RODENT ULCER

A very common form of ulceration of the skin occurring mainly in older people. The usual sites are the cheek, forehead, and bridge of the nose. Rodent ulcers cause no trouble if they are removed promptly, but if they are neglected the consequences may be serious.

If you have any kind of skin ulcer that doesn't seem to be clearing up rapidly, check with your doctor as soon as possible.

RUPTURE (HERNIA)

There are various forms of rupture or hernia.

Groin Hernia

These are very common. The characteristic feature is a rounded swelling which appears at a 'weak spot' in the abdominal wall. In one very frequent type of rupture, the swelling may extend down into the scrotum. Ruptures have nothing whatever to do with sexual function, although there is a popular myth that it does!

Some groin hernias may be related to muscular strain caused by heavy physical work, but others occur simply because there is a congenital weakness in the abdominal wall. (This is the case in all hernias encountered in babies.)

If you find a lump in the groin, see your doctor as soon as possible. Don't assume that the lump is 'just a rupture'—it might not be. In any case, all hernias need assessment by a

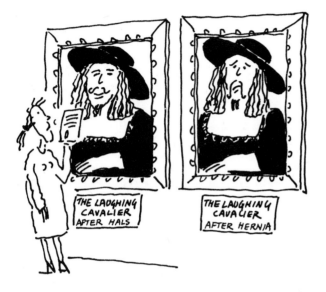

THE LAUGHING CAVALIER AFTER HALS

THE LAUGHING CAVALIER AFTER HERNIA

doctor, so please don't just buy yourself a mail-order truss (which may be totally unsuitable) or hope that the rupture will go away—it won't.

If a hernia becomes painful and tender, call the doctor at once, since it may well be 'strangulated'.

Treatment

In children, groin hernias are almost always treated by surgical operation. This produces a complete cure, and afterwards the child is normal in every way. In babies, the surgeon may decide to postpone the operation for a while until the parts are a little larger and easier to operate on.

In adults too, surgery is recommended in almost all cases. For very old, obese or infirm people, however, the surgeon may decide instead to order a properly fitted truss if he feels the patient wouldn't stand up to surgery. Very fat people are often advised to diet strictly and lose a good deal of weight. When they have done this, it may be easier to operate on them.

The operation is not a serious one, and the patient doesn't experience a lot of pain, though there is likely to be some discomfort for a week or so after surgery. If there is a rupture on both sides, the surgeon may operate on one hernia only, and postpone the repair of the other one for two or three months. This is often easier for the patient, since the discomfort after a double hernia operation can be very considerable.

After an uncomplicated hernia repair, you can expect to be out of hospital within a week or so. A few intrepid surgeons do it as a 'day case'. Light work (*i.e.* desk work, etc.) can usually be resumed within a month, but lifting weights and heavy physical activity should not be attempted for at least four months: the surgeon will give specific advice on this point in individual cases.

Because of the myth that ruptures affect virility, many patients are afraid to renew marital relations after the operation. In fact, a normal sex life can be resumed within a couple of weeks.

The most important post-operative measure which you can take in order to help yourself is to keep an eye on your weight. If you are obese, there is a greatly increased chance of recurrence of the hernia. Though this can usually be dealt with surgically, it is a nuisance to have to submit to a second operation.

In old men, the surgeon sometimes finds it difficult to repair a very large hernia without removing the testicle on that side. The patient's permission for this must always be obtained first. If the other testicle is normal, there should be no interference with the sex life, though one occasionally comes across patients who develop impotence of psychological origin as a result of worry about having lost a testicle.

Other Hernias

UMBILICAL HERNIAS. These are very common *(a)* in young children—especially West Indian babies—and *(b)* in obese adults.

If the baby has a small rupture at the navel, draw the doctor's attention to it. His advice will usually be that the swelling will disappear during the first years of life, as the child's abdominal muscles get stronger. In such cases, the only treatment that's needed is an occasional check with the doctor to see how things are progressing. The old 'treatment' of putting on binders and strapping coins over the navel has long been abandoned as useless!

If the hernia is very big or if it persists into the third or fourth year of life, surgery may be needed. The operation isn't a serious one, but it may be necessary to remove the navel altogether, which may make life a bit difficult for the child when he gets to school age. It's important for his parents to reassure him that he isn't abnormal or 'different' from his school friends.

Umbilical hernia is also frequently seen in middle-aged and elderly people who have let themselves get fat. Surgery and drastic weight reduction are indicated.

INCISIONAL HERNIAS. These are ruptures occurring through an operation scar. They are more common *(a)* where the patient is fat and *(b)* where there was infection of the original wound, resulting in delayed healing.

Surgical repair is usually possible. For obese patients, strict dieting is essential, and many pounds may have to be shed if there is to be any hope of success.

HIATUS HERNIA (*See* HIATUS HERNIA.)

S

ST VITUS' DANCE

This is the popular name for Sydenham's chorea (rheumatic chorea)—a condition which may be related to rheumatic fever, but which affects the brain rather than the joints. (*See* RHEUMATIC FEVER.) The disorder is encountered mainly in children aged seven to 15. (There is another type of chorea, called Huntington's disease, but this is a hereditary disorder appearing in later life and has no connection with rheumatic chorea.)

Rheumatic chorea is seen more often in girls than in boys. The first symptoms are restlessness and constant fidgeting. The parents may notice only that the child seems oddly clumsy. After a few days, however, it becomes apparent that one or more arms or legs are beginning to make curious writhing movements which are completely out of the child's control. At the same time, her face grimaces constantly. These symptoms disappear when she is asleep.

Phone the doctor if you suspect your child may have St Vitus' Dance. As with rheumatic fever, early treatment (and particularly rest) is essential to prevent the development of rheumatic heart disease. Recovery may take several months.

Although chorea is a disorder of certain brain centres, it does not normally affect the child's intelligence or personality.

SALPINGITIS

This is inflammation of the Fallopian tubes, which run from the ovaries to the womb. It is caused by infection with germs, and may be either acute or chronic (*i.e.* long-lasting).

Acute Salpingitis

This is a common cause of acute abdominal pain (*see* ABDOMINAL PAIN.) The chief symptoms are pain in the lower abdomen (either right-sided or left-sided, depending on which tube is involved) and fever, with a temperature of around 102°F (38.9°C). There will often have been a vaginal discharge and some menstrual irregularity in the preceding few weeks.

The patient must be admitted to hospital. With modern antibiotic treatment, the outlook is good and most people are well on the road to recovery within a couple of weeks.

Chronic Salpingitis

This is a long-standing inflammation, which may follow infection of the tubes during childbirth or abortion (miscarriage). It may sometimes be due to VD, especially where the original infection produced no symptoms (*see* GONORRHEA). Tuberculosis may also cause chronic salpingitis.

The features of this condition are variable but include intermittent pain low in the abdomen, vaginal discharge, irregular and painful periods, and sterility.

The skilled care of a gynaecologist is essential. Surgery is sometimes helpful, but prolonged medical treatment may be required.

SCABIES

A skin infection caused by a small parasite. Scabies seems to have been on the increase in recent years, and some doctors have (probably correctly) attributed this rise to the increased amount of physical contact between young people in the permissive society!

It's probably true that there is an increased chance of catching scabies under the cramped physical conditions of a pop festival, for instance. On the other hand, it could be caught on a very crowded bus or even, in my experience, in a doctor's waiting room!

The principal feature is intense itching of the skin (particularly in bed at night). This is so severe that the patient usually cannot restrain himself from tearing at his flesh. On affected areas of skin, there are small, firm, reddish bumps. These tend to be most numerous on the wrists and between the fingers, though they can also affect the armpits and genitals. The mites rarely attack the head or face.

If you have these symptoms, try to see your doctor the same day, and avoid physical contact with other people till you have had treatment. One or two applications of a special preparation which is spread over the whole body up to the neck will usually produce cure, though the itching may well take a week or two to die away completely. It's best to treat the whole family, as a rule—and certainly *both* of a pair of sexual partners.

SCALDS

These are treated in exactly the same way as burns (*see* BURNS in the A–Z of Emergencies.)

SCARS

Ugly scars following injury, burns or surgery can be a problem. If they cannot be disguised by a cosmetic preparation of the Covermark or Boots brand type, plastic surgery may be helpful.

Not all cases are suitable, however, and there are some people whose skins respond to almost any kind of cut (including the most careful surgical incision) by forming a mass of raised, smooth tissue called a 'keloid'; this is a particular problem among black patients. Operation on keloids is a very specialized business indeed, and should never be undertaken without a great deal of thought. The patient should discuss carefully with the surgeon whether it is worth running the risk of making things worse.

SCARLET FEVER (SCARLATINA)

This used to be a very common, serious disease. At the beginning of this century, it killed many children each year.

Nowadays, for some unknown reason, scarlet fever is not very common and rarely serious. It often consists only of a sore throat and a rash. Treated promptly and carefully with modern drugs, it is not likely to produce complications.

The disorder is basically a sensitivity to a toxin produced by the streptococcus germ, an organism which is a widespread cause of sore throats, tonsillitis and other infections. Most people who have a 'strep throat' are better within a few days. In scarlet fever, however, the initial sore throat or tonsillitis is followed by a curious pink rash, made up of tiny scarlet spots.

In the initial stage, the child's only symptoms are those of either a sore throat infection or acute tonsillitis (*see* TONSILS AND TONSILLITIS). Such symptoms may be a raised temperature, vomiting, cough, and hoarseness.

One or two days later, the rash appears—first behind the ears, and then spreading over the face and the whole body. Characteristically, the area round the mouth is spared and remains pale in comparison with the rest of the skin. The tongue usually has a white fur on it, but this later peels off, often leaving a red 'strawberry-like' appearance.

Your child will have treatment with penicillin (or sometimes other drugs) and should recover within 10 days or so. Because of the slight risk of kidney complications, he should be under the doctor's care for about three weeks after recovery, and he will need at least one urine examination at the lab.

Incubation and Quarantine

The incubation period of scarlet fever is very short (two to seven days) but in this particular disease this information is not of much value, since it is only very rarely that a child will have caught the infection from someone with scarlet fever. It is far more likely to have come from some completely unidentifiable person with, say, a sore throat of some other streptococcal infection.

The quarantine period from the onset of the disorder should be determined by the doctor in charge of the case. Some doctors still prefer a quarantine of three weeks, but others feel this is overlong these days, since the chances of passing scarlet fever to another child are small. Schools still tend to get a bit alarmed about the diagnosis of scarlet fever, however, and it's best to get an 'all-clear' certificate before the child goes back.

SCHIZOPHRENIA

A very common form of mental illness (*see* MENTAL ILLNESS), which probably affects at the very least 30 million people in the world.

Schizophrenia does not, as so many people think, mean 'split personality', in the 'Dr. Jekyll and Mr. Hyde' sense. It means disintegration of the personality, with partial or total withdrawal from reality. There may be delusions and hallucinations, and admission to a psychiatric hospital is usually necessary.

There is no point in describing the early features of schizophrenia in detail, but if a young person aged between 15 and 20 shows disturbing mental symptoms which amount to more than the apathy and vagueness which is to be expected from time to time in the young, then contact your family doctor. From a short chat with the young person, he should be able to form a reasonable conclusion as to whether anything is really wrong.

If schizophrenia is diagnosed, the outlook, while serious, is not so bleak as it used to be. New methods of treatment, and particularly the powerful phenothiazine tranquillizers, have revolutionized the position. Mental hospitals which were packed full of hundreds of schizophrenics are at last beginning to empty. A good many patients these days can truly be described as cured, while many others, with the help of daily drug treatment and the encouragement and support of their families, can lead reasonably happy and useful lives.

SCIATICA

Sciatica *isn't* a disease or a medical condition in itself. The word simply means pain running down the back of the leg, from the lower spine or the buttock to the calf. It is made worse by raising the leg straight in the air while lying down.

The presence of sciatica means that something is wrong in or around the lower part of the spine, where the nerves running to the leg emerge from the spinal cord.

There are several conditions which can cause this kind of pain, so full investigation, including X-ray of the lower spine, may be necessary. Among the most common causes is a prolapsed lumbar disc (*see* **'Slipped' Disc**, under BACKACHE).

SCURVY

Scurvy is the disease caused by deficiency of vitamin C, the vitamin found in fresh fruit and green vegetables.

Scurvy used to be very common indeed among sailors on long voyages. In the 18th century, the Scots naval surgeon James Lynd was able to eradicate the disease from the Royal Navy by introducing limes into the sailor's daily diet. (It's said that this is why Americans took to calling the English 'Limeys'.)

Nowadays, scurvy is almost unknown among adults, but it can occur in infants. The first symptoms include intense pain in the bones of the legs, and bleeding from the gums. The disease usually appears between the ages of six and 18 months, and is rare in breast-fed babies, because mother's milk contains far more vitamin C than artificial milk.

Nevertheless, babies should have vitamin C supplements, *e.g.* in the form of orange juice (which should not be boiled or heated—this will destroy the vitamin). This should be continued up to about the age of four. Make sure also that, when your child goes onto a mixed diet, he gets plenty of oranges, grapefruit, tomatoes, lettuce etc. If you do this, the risk of scurvy is practically nil.

SEA-SICKNESS (*See* TRAVEL SICKNESS.)

SEBACEOUS CYST

A very common form of cystic swelling in the skin. The old name for a sebaceous cyst is a 'wen', and one still sometimes hears country people use this term. Most sebaceous cysts occur on the scalp or face. Removal is usually a fairly straightforward procedure. The operation is carried out under local anaesthetic and any scar left should be small.

SEXUAL DIFFICULTIES (*See* INTERCOURSE—DIFFICULTIES IN, and IMPOTENCE.)

SHINGLES

Known medically as *herpes zoster*, this is a common and often trying disease. It is caused by the same virus which is responsible for chicken-pox, and adults may catch shingles from a child with the latter condition. The virus attacks one or more nerve roots, and the first result of this is pain in the area of skin supplied by the particular nerve involved.

A day or two later, this strip of skin becomes covered by a red, blistery rash, which may be itchy as well as painful. The rash and the pain slowly pass off, usually over a period of several weeks.

The commonest sites for shingles are the sides of the chest and abdomen. Where the eye or ear are involved, however, the problem is more serious, and it may well be necessary for the doctor to call in a specialist, particularly when the sight is threatened.

If the diagnosis is made *early*, there is a chance of terminating the attack with Herpid—a fairly new anti-viral 'paint'. Other new anti-virals are on the way, but they too will have to be applied right at the outset of the disease.

Later on, however, there is no specific treatment for the shingles virus. Aspirin or other pain-killing tablets are helpful in relieving both pain and irritation. Many doctors recommend calamine lotion or collodion for application to the skin, and some prescribe olive oil when the blisters dry up and the scabs start to come away.

Neuralgia may sometimes persist for many months after an attack of shingles, particularly in elderly people. Powerful pain-killers may be needed, and some doctors prescribe electrical stimulation to the affected area. Simple rubbing with the finger-tips is also helpful. (*See also* NEURALGIA).

The patient's family should keep a look out for the severe depression which the pain sometimes induces. It is all too easy for an elderly person who has been in agony for weeks or months to become suicidal. If symptoms of depression appear, always ask the doctor to see the patient. (*See also* DEPRESSION.)

SHOCK

People who have suffered serious injury (for instance, in a road accident) may go into shock immediately afterwards. This is particularly likely where there is internal or external bleeding.

The shocked patient feels faint or light-headed, and may collapse. He usually goes very pale, and his skin becomes clammy and cold. He may break into a sweat or shiver. His pulse is likely to be fast and 'thready', and he may gasp for air.

First aid

Lie the patient down, preferably with the lower part of

his body slightly raised. Control any bleeding, as described under the heading BLEEDING in the A–Z of Emergencies.

Reassure the patient, and make him as comfortable as you can. Don't let him sit up, even if he becomes restless. Cover him with a light sheet or blanket to keep him reasonably warm. Don't give him anything by mouth, even if he complains of thirst (often a prominent feature of shock).

Get him to hospital by ambulance (or lying flat in the back of a car) as soon as you can. *Delay may be fatal, especially where shock is due to internal bleeding.*

Note: It used to be taught that the correct first aid for a patient in shock was to heat him up (for instance, with hot-water bottles, etc.) and give him hot sweet tea or coffee by mouth. This advice is now known to be wrong, so *don't* use these measures!

SICKLE CELL ANAEMIA

A form of anaemia (*see* ANAEMIA) found only in those of African descent. The condition is due to an abnormal gene (or hereditary factor) which is thought to be carried by approximately 10% of people in West Africa and the West Indies, and probably by roughly the same proportion of black people in the USA and in Britain.

These 'carriers' are perfectly healthy, except that they seem to run a slightly increased risk of suffering from an unusual type of bleeding from the kidney.

When two 'carriers' marry, however, some of their children may well have sickle cell anaemia. In addition to the ordinary symptoms of a low blood count—tiredness and breathlessness—children who are 'sicklers' are liable to jaundice and to episodes of severe pain, especially joint pain, which may be mistaken for rheumatic fever or some other condition. Their growth is likely to be very stunted.

The outlook in sickle cell anaemia was very poor until recent years, but new methods of treatment have made a considerable difference to the sickler's life. Therapy should, if possible, be undertaken by a hospital unit with considerable experience of dealing with this problem.

SILICOSIS

This is a type of pneumoconiosis (*see* PNEUMOCONIOSIS) which is seen in brick workers, in foundry workers, in miners who are involved in rock-drilling, and in various other occupational groups who are exposed to silica dust.

SINUSITIS

Inflammation of the air sinuses which lie in the front part of the skull, above and around the nose. There are two sinuses in the forehead, two behind the cheeks, and two behind the bridge of the nose. Other sinuses lie farther back, behind the eyes.

All these cavities drain into the nose through small openings. When there's a cold in the nose, it's quite easy for infection to spread into the sinuses. If this happens, the sinus lining may swell up and block the opening. Pus which forms inside the cavity therefore can't drain away.

The result is intense pain over the sinus involved. Other features of sinusitis include fever and an unpleasant blocked-up feeling in the head. There may also be an intermittent discharge of pus down the back of the nose, and into the throat and lungs.

If you are prone to sinusitis, see your doctor at the first sign of an attack, because it may be possible to cut the infection short at this stage. The doctor will usually prescribe treatment with antibiotics and decongestants. Aspirin and other analgesics are useful too. You'll find that you get better more quickly if you try to stay in a moist, dust-free, and reasonably warm atmosphere until the infection is over. Steam inhalations are very useful.

Some patients with recurrent sinusitis benefit from surgery, and all patients who have had several attacks should be assessed by an ear, nose and throat surgeon.

SKIN DISORDERS (*See* ACNE, ATHLETE'S FOOT, BARBER'S ITCH, BOILS, CARBUNCLES, ECZEMA, ERYSIPELAS, PIMPLES, PSORIASIS, RINGWORM, RODENT ULCER, SCABIES, and URTICARIA.)

SLEEPLESSNESS (*See* INSOMNIA.)

SLIMMING (*See* FATNESS.)

'SLIPPED' DISC (*See under* BACKACHE.)

SMALLPOX

An infectious disease, caused by a virus. Once one of the world's worst scourges, it's now believed to have vanished.

The last known outbreak occurred some years ago, when smallpox germs escaped from a research lab in Birmingham. The only real danger today seems to be that a related jungle infection called 'monkeypox' might change its nature and become more like smallpox.

Features of smallpox include headache, fever, and often vomiting. These precede the appearance of the rash by about three to four days. The rash is much like that of chicken-pox, but is thicker on the upper part of the face and on the arms and legs than it is on the trunk.

The incubation period of smallpox was usually about 10 to 16 days. Quarantine was usually about 17 days. There is, of course, no need now for your children to have smallpox vaccination—specially as it carries risks of its own.

SMOKING (*See* TOBACCO.)

SNAKE BITE
There are 2,500 known species of snake, and less than a tenth of these are venomous. Snake bites in most Western countries are unlikely to kill an adult, though immediate medical attention should always be sought. There is greater risk of death occurring where the patient is a young child.

If the snake has been killed, take it with you for identification. Unless you are a first-aider skilled in treating snake bite, leave the wound alone. Don't put on tourniquets or carry out the traditional cowboy remedy of cutting into the skin and trying to suck out the poison—you are likely to make things worse if you don't know what you are doing. Just keep the patient calm, and get him to medical help as fast as you can. If he collapses, you may have to give the 'kiss of life' as described under FIRST AID TECHNIQUES OF RESUSCITATION in the A–Z of Emergencies.

In French and Italian mountain regions, walkers are advised to take anti-snake venom injections with them in case of a bite, and this is an excellent idea.

SNORING
There's no easy remedy for snoring, though a child who

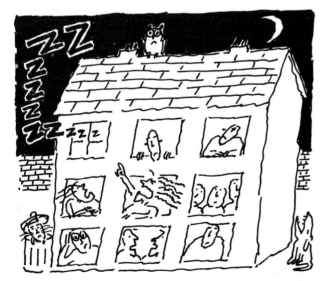

snores persistently may possibly need his adenoids removed. In adults, the only remedy for the aggrieved spouse is to keep elbowing the snorer until he or she rolls onto his or her side! This usually terminates the noise, because it's very hard to snore except when lying on the back.

Some wives stitch objects such as clothes brushes on the backs of their husbands' nightwear to discourage lying in the snoring position. If all else fails, earplugs may help.

SORE THROAT
Sore throat, or pharyngitis, is a very common disorder, and most people get it at least once or twice a year. The condition usually occurs with much greater frequency among smokers, and if you have several bouts of pharyngitis each winter, you'd do better to give up cigarettes.

Most cases of sore throat in children and other non-smokers are due to infection with either viruses, or bacteria. Viruses don't respond to antibiotics, so it's usually reasonable to try the effect of aspirin and hot salt water gargles alone for 24 hours before you consult the doctor. (*See also* QUINSY, TONSILS and TONSILLITIS.)

SPASTIC DISORDERS
Babies who have suffered brain damage (especially at birth) may develop what's called 'cerebral palsy'. Lay people often call these children 'spastic', and the term is a convenient one, though it's not entirely accurate, since spasticity (that is, increased tone) of the limbs is not present in all cases.

These unfortunate children may have many disabilities to cope with. Their speech may be hard to understand, and they may have poor control of their limbs. Their faces may grimace constantly, and this contorted appearance may lead the observer to think that a spastic child is mentally deficient or in some way deranged.

Of course, this isn't so. Many children with cerebral palsy have perfectly normal minds and high intelligence—there was, for instance, an Irishman with this disorder who grew up to be a best-selling novelist.

It's very important, therefore, for the child's parents, brothers, sisters, and friends to treat him as normally as possible. He should be allowed to join in games and almost any other kind of children's activities without being 'molly-coddled'. If he can go to a normal school, that's fine, since it will help him not to feel isolated and 'different'. Even if he has to go to a special school for handicapped children, he should be encouraged to mix with as many friends as possible out of school hours.

Some hospitals have cerebral palsy units these days, and it's helpful if a child can be seen fairly regularly at this kind of specialized centre. The doctor in charge will advise about the possibility of getting assistance from local social workers with a particular interest in spastic children and their problems.

Most parents derive considerable benefit from joining the associations (*e.g.* the Spastics Society, 12 Park Crescent, London W1; tel: 01-636 5020) which mothers and fathers of children with cerebral palsy have founded in several countries. Not only do these associations provide practical help, but they have the great advantage that they enable parents to realize that they are not alone in the difficulties they are facing.

SPOTS (*See* PIMPLES.)

SPRAINS

A sprain occurs when a joint is forced beyond its normal range of movement. This tears fibres of the ligaments or tendons around the joint, and the result is moderately severe pain which is made worse by any movement that puts the torn ligament or tendon on the stretch. There may also be bruising and swelling. The joints most commonly affected by sprains are the ankle, wrist and knee.

First Aid

PR Spray (which many sports clubs etc. have in their first aid bags) is useful in providing at least some pain relief. Lie the patient down if he feels faint. Remove any constricting shoes, socks, tights, bracelets, etc.—if the part swells up, it may be impossible to take them off later on.

Rest the joint in the most comfortable position. A wad of cotton wool soaked in cold water will usually give some relief of pain. If you know how to apply a bandage properly, do so—this will keep the swelling down. It's best if you use a broad bandage, firmly applied over a thick layer of cotton wool. If it's the wrist, elbow or shoulder which has been sprained, support the arm with a sling.

In general, try to *elevate* the part so that fluid drains away from it. If you have some *ice* available, put it in a cloth bag or a facecloth and gently rub it on the skin over the affected part.

Always make sure the patient goes to a doctor. It may save time with a severe sprain to go directly to a hospital Accident Department, since an X-ray will be required to rule out a fracture.

SPUTUM

There's a tendency for smokers to regard a bit of morning sputum (phlegm) as being 'normal'. This brilliant idea is wrong! Smoker or not, if you are coughing up sputum, you ought to see a doctor, and particularly if you have been producing it for more than a week, or if the material is green, yellow, pink or blood-stained. Blood-stained sputum (haemoptysis) always needs investigation, including a chest X-ray.

SQUINT

In an adult, the sudden development of a squint needs immediate investigation, preferably by a neurologist.

In young babies, slight crossing of the eyes is very common. In the first three months of life, this symptom does not matter, provided that it only occurs momentarily. If it's there a lot of the time, have a doctor examine the child.

Similarly, any apparent squint present after the age of three months needs medical assessment. The condition may well be of no significance, but let your doctor decide. If an actual disorder of the eye muscles might be present, he'll send the child to an eye specialist right away.

Don't put off having something done about a baby's crossed eyes. Even the most serious squint can be treated successfully by glasses and/or operation, but leaving things alone can do irreparable damage to the sight.

STAMMERING

A stammer or stutter isn't usually due to physical disease but is related to emotional factors. Slight stammering is common in the two- to three-year-old age group, but in most cases it passes off completely, particularly if the parents do something about whatever is upsetting the toddler.

Factors which may provoke a stammer in a child include worries about whether his parents love him. He may be upset by the arrival of a new baby, or disturbed by family quarrels. Sometimes, he is naturally left-handed, and the parents' attempts to 'correct' him to right-handedness seem to start him stammering. In such cases, he should be allowed completely free choice as to which hand he uses.

If a child's stammer persists to the age of three or four, it's best to consult the family doctor. In severe cases, speech therapy will be necessary.

A new but expensive device—the 'Edinburgh masker'—is helpful, because it stops the patient hearing his own nervous attempts at speech and therefore stops his stammering.

STERILITY

About 10 to 15% of marriages have trouble with fertility. Inability to have children is a very distressing problem for any couple. Of course, not everyone can expect to have children exactly whenever they want them, but if you've been trying for, say, 12 months without success, then it's as well to seek help.

The family doctor will usually refer patients to a gynaecologist who specializes in the treatment of infertility; many hospitals run regular infertility clinics these days.

At these clinics, the first problem is sometimes found to be that the wife is still a virgin and the couple are not really having intercourse at all! This may sound astonishing, but even in these supposedly well-informed days there are a surprising number of husbands and wives who simply don't know how to set about having a child (though they usually think that whatever they are doing is how babies are made).

Assuming that this problem does not apply, however, the next thing is to decide whether the couple are trying at the right time of the month—*i.e.* ovulation, which is usually about 14 days before the start of a period. The subject of the conception day is discussed more fully in the section **Ovulation and Periods** (under the heading PERIOD PROBLEMS). If you have intercourse each day for three or four days running at about the time of ovulation, then the chances of pregnancy are much better.

If this fails, full investigation of both parties is necessary. Even today, men tend to blame infertility on women, but the fact is that in many marriages it's the husband who is sterile, even though he may be potent or indeed highly virile.

The gynaecologist will therefore arrange a lab test on the husband's seminal fluid, mainly to see how many sperms it contains, and if the individual sperms are active and normally formed.

A post-coital test is also useful. The wife is examined shortly after intercourse, and a check is made as to whether the husband's sperms are surviving in the secretions of the vagina and cervix.

The wife also needs full investigation, of course. She may have to have a D and C (dilation and curettage), or scrape of the womb lining. Very often, the specialist will test whether her Fallopian tubes (which carry the eggs, or ova, from the ovaries to the womb) are blocked or not. This is checked by a simple procedure in which a little carbon dioxide gas is blown through the tubes from a narrow catheter inserted into the vagina. X-rays of the tubes can be carried out by injecting a radio-opaque dye in the same way. Both these procedures are more comfortable under general anaesthesia, but they can also be performed without an anaesthetic. And the newish technique of laparoscopy (in which a slim telescope-like device is used to inspect the internal organs) can be of great help in investigating infertility.

Treatment

If some disorder of the female genital tract is present, it can often be treated satisfactorily, and pregnancy may follow within a few months. If the Fallopian tubes are blocked, however, there may be a considerable problem, though some surgeons are beginning to achieve encouraging results with Fallopian tube surgery.

And of course, Mr Steptoe and Dr Edwards and others in Australia and elsewhere have achieved a number of 'test tube babies'—babies who are conceived in a laboratory dish from the husband's sperm and the wife's 'egg' or ovum. The fertilized ovum is then put into the womb *from below* —thereby by-passing the diseased or missing tube.

In many cases of female infertility, particularly those linked with hormone imbalance, the new 'fertility drugs' may be very helpful.

Where infertility is due to the husband, the outlook is not usually very hopeful, though there are ways of raising low sperm counts. If there is no prospect of his fathering a child, he and his wife should consider whether they want to have a baby by AID (artificial insemination by donor). An increasing number of gynaecologists are willing to arrange this procedure, and couples who have chosen it are usually very happy with their baby.

Adoption is the obvious alternative—if you can find a baby to adopt.

STERILIZATION

(For male sterilization, *see* VASECTOMY.)

A good many women nowadays undergo sterilization by means of a fairly simple operation which involves tying off or cutting the two Fallopian tubes (which carry the ova, or eggs, from the ovaries to the womb).

This operation has no effect at all on sexual function, or on the periods, and doesn't lead to menopausal symptoms. (I should add that there *is* a theory that it can lead to heavier periods. But this is far from proven.) Often it can be done by just pushing two instruments through the wall of the tummy, and recovery is very rapid after this 'laparoscopic' operation.

It's important for the patient and her husband to be really sure that they want sterilization done, however. Sterilization *can* sometimes be reversed, but it's a difficult and uncertain procedure which many surgeons quite understandably won't undertake. It's best, therefore, to assume that the operation is once and for all.

STILL'S DISEASE

This is basically a childhood form of rheumatoid arthritis

(*see* RHEUMATOID ARTHRITIS). It usually arises between the ages of two and nine, and may 'burn itself out' by adulthood. The features include joint pain and stiffness, stunting of growth, and eye troubles. Judicious treatment with drugs such as aspirin, gold, steroids and ACTH, as well as physiotherapy and sometimes surgery, will give good results in many cases nowadays.

It's often a good idea if the child can have treatment from a specialized hospital unit devoted largely to the care of patient's with Still's disease. The parents shouldn't regard the child as an invalid, but should encourage him to lead a full, active and happy life, as far as possible.

STONES
People are sometimes alarmed at being told they have stones, but in fact it's quite common for these *calculi* (as they are called medically) to form in various sites within the body, notably in the gall bladder and in the kidney (*see* GALL BLADDER and KIDNEY in the A–Z of Parts of the Body). Stones may also be found in the bladder, though this is not as common in temperate countries as it is in the Middle and Far East.

Stones containing calcium will show up on ordinary X-rays. It may not be possible to diagnose other stones except by special X-ray procedures which involve the injection of radio-opaque dye.

Some calculi (for instance gall stones which are producing no symptoms) do not necessarily require operation, but most stones should be removed surgically without delay.

STRICTURE
This term is applied to a narrowing of the urinary passage in men. A stricture causes difficulty in passing urine, and often acute retention (*see* RETENTION OF URINE). Surgical treatment of stricture involves widening the urinary passage with special dilators.

STROKES
Strokes, or cerebro-vascular accidents (CVAs), can occur in several ways.

Types of Stroke
CEREBRAL HAEMORRHAGE. This happens when a blood vessel breaks inside the skull and bleeding into the brain follows, with resulting destruction of brain tissue.
CEREBRAL THROMBOSIS. This happens when a clot (or thrombosis) blocks a blood vessel inside the skull. Again, brain tissue dies because it is starved of oxygen.
CEREBRAL EMBOLISM. This happens when material from

elsewhere in the body (for instance, a clot coming from the heart) passes up into the skull and blocks a blood vessel, with effects broadly similar to those of cerebral thrombosis.

Symptoms of a Stroke
These vary quite a bit, and the symptoms of a minor stroke may amount to no more than a slight vagueness or transient speech difficulty. The commonest occurrence in a major stroke is that the patient becomes paralyzed in one arm and one leg. One side of the face may also be affected, and if the patient remains conscious the speech is often severely impaired.

First Aid
Lie the stroke victim on his side, remove any false teeth, and loosen the clothing at the neck. If the patient is unconscious, treat him as described under UNCONSCIOUSNESS. If he is conscious, simply make him as comfortable as possible until the doctor arrives. Remember that the confused or unconscious patient will be very bewildered when he comes round. Even though he cannot speak, he may well be able to hear and understand you, so try to reassure him as much as possible.

Aftercare
The patient who recovers from a minor stroke will probably be completely healthy in every way. After a major stroke, however, there may be a very considerable degree of disability. Help in the way of physiotherapy and occupational therapy can be of the greatest importance to the stroke patient. Visits once or twice a week to a special unit where patients are retrained to cope with the difficulties of dressing, washing, etc., are of inestimable value. Ask your doctor what facilities are available in your area.

If high blood pressure is present, this will probably need lifelong treatment (*see* BLOOD PRESSURE).

Finally, the support and encouragement of his own family is absolutely vital to the stroke victim. It's all too easy when one is old and paralyzed down one side to give up hope altogether. This should not be allowed to happen if at all possible.

STUTTERING (*See* STAMMERING.)

STYES
These are infections of the hair follicles from which the eyelashes grow, caused by the same germs that are responsible for boils, carbuncles, and many septic 'spots'.

If you develop a stye, bathe the eye with cotton wool

soaked in hot water. (*Warning*: be careful how you dispose of the cotton wool, which will be infected by germs from the stye.)

If a head forms on the stye, you can release the pus by plucking out the eyelash, preferably with tweezers. Bathe the eye and wash your hands (and the tweezers) very carefully afterwards. Antiseptic eye ointment will help to prevent the spread of infection.

If you get recurrent styes, see your doctor and have a test for diabetes.

Note: No one with a stye should be allowed to prepare food in a factory or restaurant until the infection has cleared up.

SUB-ARACHNOID HAEMORRHAGE
A condition in which bleeding occurs within the skull as a result of weakness in a blood vessel. The condition is not uncommonly seen in youngish men. Typically, the patient collapses, complaining of a feeling like a sudden blow on the back of the ear. He may rapidly become unconscious. He must, of course, be transferred to hospital as soon as possible.

The outlook for recovery is quite good. In some patients, it is possible to operate in order to make good the weakness of the blood vessel within the skull. If raised blood pressure is present, this will need long-term treatment (*see* BLOOD PRESSURE).

SUICIDE (*See under* DEPRESSION.)

SUNBURN AND SUNSTROKE
Both these conditions are avoidable, provided that you remember the golden rule, which is: treat the sun with respect.

Every year, quite a number of people who go seeking the sun make themselves ill through overexposure to its rays. Even if the resort you go to is only a couple of hundred miles nearer the equator than your home, the sun's rays there are going to be less filtered-off and more powerful than you and your family are used to.

It's common for doctors who practise at the seaside, even in Britain, to be called in to see children who have arrived a couple of days before and been allowed to go out and play all day long in the sun without a hat or a shirt. The result may be severe sunburn or, perhaps more commonly, a splitting headache, a slight temperature, and an off-colour feeling that ruins the next few days for the whole family.

So, take things easy. In Victorian and Edwardian days, Englishmen who went to the South of France had a rule that on the first day they would expose only their feet to the

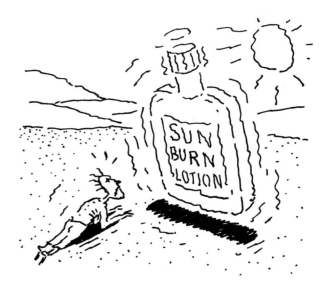

sun, on the second day their feet and shins, on the third, their feet, shins and knees, and so on. Well, perhaps such extreme caution isn't really all that necessary (particularly if you're on a one week package tour to Spain or the Bahamas) but the basic idea was right—take things easy, unless you want to land up in hospital.

Use plenty of a good protective lotion or cream before you lie down on the beach. Para-aminobenzoic acid (PABA) preparations are particularly effective screening agents. Avoid the midday sun.

Be wary about going to sleep in the sun, especially without a hat—you may wake up frazzled. In tropical and subtropical climates, it may be dangerous to go snorkelling for long periods with just a swimsuit on—the sun's rays, beating through the water, will still burn your back. Many experienced snorkellers, particularly those with fair skins, always wear a light shirt while in the water.

Treatment
SUNBURN. Mild sunburn can be treated with any of the proprietary soothing creams. Many people favour calamine lotion, but others find that this stops the skin from 'breathing', and so increases the intense itching which often goes with sunburn.

The most effective pain-killing preparations are those which contain a mild local anaesthetic, for instance Solarcaine. These have only recently gone on sale in the UK, however, presumably because of fears that people might use them to kill the pain and then carry on getting more and more seriously burned. In practice, few people are silly enough to do this. But local anaesthetic preparations can cause serious skin reactions sometimes.

SUNSTROKE. This is rare outside the very hot regions of the world. Get the patient into the shade, keep him lying down and comfortable, and stay with him till medical help arrives. However thirsty he is, don't give him *large* quantities of water or other fluids to drink: this is very dangerous. It's best to restrict him to a sip of water (or, if available, water with a little salt added) every 15 minutes or so. Thirst and dryness of the lips can be alleviated to some extent by gently wiping the mouth with a damp cloth.

SYPHILIS

The most serious of the venereal diseases (*see* VENEREAL DISEASES). Fortunately, it's far less common nowadays in Britain that it used to be, and other types of VD (for instance, gonorrhea and NSU) are more frequently encountered. Promiscuous homosexuals are at risk, however.

Syphilis is caused by a germ called *Treponema pallidum*. It can always be cured, if it's caught in the early stages. If it's not properly treated, however, the long-term consequences (which include insanity and death) are quite horrifying. Fortunately such late complications rarely occur these days, partly because most people have the sense to go to a doctor or 'Special Clinic' as soon as the symptoms appear. A few patients are still unwise enough to think that the disease will go away by itself—but it won't.

Symptoms

Syphilis is acquired by having sex (though not necessarily actual intercourse) with an infected person. (*N.B.* In many countries, though not in all, there is a very high risk of infection in having sex with prostitutes.) Very occasionally, a person with a syphilis sore on the lip may infect others simply by kissing.

The first symptom occurs about a month after exposure. A firm, painless sore develops on the genitals (or sometimes on other parts of the body, *e.g.* the lip or nipple). In women, there is a danger that the sore may sometimes be too far inside to be noticed.

The sore is usually about the size of your fingernail. A small amount of discharge may come from it. The nearby groin glands will probably swell up. After a variable period of time, the sore will go away. This does not mean the disease is cured—it isn't.

In the secondary stage of syphilis, which is usually a few weeks later, there may be a spell of general ill health, with sore throat, skin rashes, mouth ulcers and fever.

The tertiary (late) stage of syphilis occurs years later. Its appalling effects on the brain, heart and other organs need not be described here. These complications will *not* occur if you have sought treatment in the early stages of the disease.

Treatment and Prevention

Patients are sometimes tempted to treat themselves with 'borrowed' drugs because they are embarrassed about going to the doctor, but this is foolish—treatment is a specialized business. If it is to be adequate, proper lab tests have to be carried out.

In order to obtain these tests, you really need to attend the confidential 'Special Clinic' at your nearest large hospital. You will probably be given a course of treatment lasting approximately two weeks, and it's vital that you don't abandon it part of the way through. You'll also be asked to return for further tests at a later date, and you'll be given printed cards to hand or send to anyone you have slept with.

It should go without saying that anyone who has syphilis (or any other form of VD) should on no account have sex with anybody until they are cured.

T

TB (*See* TUBERCULOSIS.)

TEMPERATURE (RAISED OR LOW)

The normal body temperature is about 98.4°F to 98.6°F (36.9°C to 37.0°C), but slight variations are of no significance. Most doctors are familiar with the very occasional patient who summons medical help when his temperature is 'nearly up to 99, doctor!'

Nobody's temperature stays fixed at 'normal'. Particularly in children, the temperature moves up and down by as much as a degree Farenheit in the course of the day. All sorts of factors, including the weather, affect the body temperature. In women, it's variable at different times of the 'month' (*see* **Ovulation and Periods** under PERIOD PROBLEMS.)

What temperature indicates that 'something's wrong'? Well, in adults a reading of over 99.5°F (37.5°C) indicates that something is probably amiss, though it may be as trivial as a cold.

In young children, a reading of over 100°F (37.8°C) usually

indicates some sort of illness (again, possibly very trivial), though an excited toddler can easily push his temperature up to this level for a short time by running about or crying, particularly if he is warmly wrapped up.

At what level of temperature should you call the doctor? It's quite impossible to give a firm rule about this. If in doubt, phone your doctor, describe the child's symptoms and tell him what the thermometer reading is; he'll decide whether a visit is necessary.

Causes of an Abnormal Temperature

LOW TEMPERATURES. These are unusual, except where someone has been exposed to cold for an excessive period of time. This condition of hypothermia is seen in premature babies (*see* PREMATURITY in the A–Z of Emergencies) who haven't been wrapped up warmly enough, in walkers or climbers suffering from exposure, and (very commonly) in old people whose houses have inadequate heating. If anyone's temperature appears to be below 96.5°F (35.8°C), put the thermometer back in the mouth for another two minutes. If the reading is still below this level, wrap the patient in warm blankets and contact the doctor.

HIGH TEMPERATURE. As we've said above, a normal baby or toddler can have a slightly raised temperature when he's been active or crying. Otherwise, a high temperature is almost always due to infection of some sort. The commonest causes are:

in children—colds and other virus infections, tonsilitis, ear infections (*otitis media*), chest infections (*e.g.* bronchitis and pneumonia), kidney infection (pyelitis), gastro-enteritis, appendicitis, mumps, measles, chicken-pox, German measles, and whooping cough;

in adults—colds, influenza and other virus infections, sore throat, laryngitis, chest infections, kidney infection (pyelitis) and glandular fever (infectious mononucleosis).

There are also rarer causes of fever, including a very large number of tropical diseases.

Treatment of Raised Temperature

Don't start treatment with penicillin or any other antibiotic you happen to have left over in the medicine cupboard. In the case of a child with a high temperature, the main thing is to cool the patient down a bit. You can do this in several ways:

(i) by giving aspirin or similar preparations;

(ii) by getting rid of unnecessary blankets and clothing, which only help to keep the temperature up;

(iii) by turning down room heating until the atmosphere is cool;

(iv) by sponging the body with tepid water—this should always be done where a child with a temperature has had a convulsion (*see* CONVULSIONS in A–Z of Emergencies);

(v) by giving iced drinks.

How to Take the Temperature

A lot of people don't know how to take a temperature. Everyone should be able to carry out this simple procedure.

The first thing, of course, is to buy or borrow a thermometer. Every family (and particularly every family with children) ought to have one, and they cost very little in relation to their usefulness. It will help your doctor considerably, if, when you phone him about an illness, you are able to give the temperature.

Having got your thermometer, have a good look at it. If it's an old Farenheit one, it'll be marked from about 94°F to about 107°F. The degrees are usually divided up into fifths, each of which is 0.2°F. At the 'Normal' mark, there's usually an arrow, or the letter 'N', or both. The new *Centigrade* thermometers tend to run from about 35°C to about 41°C, with the N or the arrow at about 37°C.

Before using the thermometer, make sure the mercury is down below the lower end of the scale. If it isn't, shake it down. You do this by holding the upper end of the thermometer (the one away from the bulb) and snapping the instrument sharply downwards three or four times with a firm, wristy action. This is easy with a little practice.

Where possible, always take the temperature in the mouth, with the bulb under the tongue. All temperatures given in this book and most others are mouth readings. With a baby

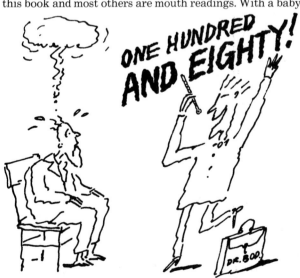

or toddler, however, you'll have to use the armpit—hold the child's arm gently but firmly across his tummy so that the bulb in his armpit is kept warm.

Armpit temperatures are slightly lower than mouth ones (usually about a degree Farenheit or so), but if you're telling the doctor your child's temperature, don't add on a bit for this—you'll only cause confusion. Simply tell him you've given him an armpit temperature, and not a mouth one.

Don't try to take a child's temperature by putting the thermometer in the rectum. This method used to be widely employed until not long ago, but occasional nasty accidents do occur with it, particularly in the newborn. The armpit is completely safe and very convenient.

Though the thermometer may sometimes be marked 'half minute', always leave it in place for at least two minutes.

After taking the temperature, shake the thermometer down as before. Wash it in soap and water (cold water!) and return it to its case. If the patient is likely to be suffering from infection, it's a good idea instead to stand the thermometer in a little jar of mild disinfectant until you need to take his temperature again.

TETANUS (*See* LOCKJAW)

THROAT, SORE (*See* SORE THROAT.)

THROMBOSIS

Thrombosis means clot (or thrombus) formation.
For cerebral thrombosis, *see* STROKE.
For coronary thrombosis, *see* CORONARY THROMBOSIS.

Vein Thrombosis

SUPERFICIAL VEIN THROMBOSIS. This is thrombosis occurring in a vein running just under the skin. It is common and usually of trivial importance. This kind of thrombosis may occur in association with phlebitis (vein inflammation), or following an intravenous blood transfusion or other infusion. It may also be deliberately induced as part of a treatment for varicose veins. (*See also* PHLEBITIS and VARICOSE VEINS.)

All that happens in a superficial thrombosis is that the vein becomes painful and hard, and feels like a tender cord under the skin. The doctor may prescribe anti-inflammatory drugs and a firm bandage. Normal activity is usually allowed.

DEEP VEIN THROMBOSIS. Thrombosis in a deep vein of the leg or one of the veins of the pelvis may be serious, since a piece of the clot may break off into the vein and pass to the lungs, causing the common disorder known as pulmonary embolism. The subject is discussed further under the heading PULMONARY EMBOLISM.

THRUSH

Also known as Monilia or Candida, thrush is a fungus which very frequently infects human beings at various sites. The two organs most commonly affected are the mouth and the vagina, but it also hits the skin and nails.

Oral Thrush

Thrush infection of the mouth occurs mainly in babies and is characterized by the appearance of multiple white patches on the membrane inside the cheeks and on the tongue. It almost looks as though little flecks of milk had been left inside the baby's mouth. Underneath the patches, however, the delicate membrane is inflamed and sore, and the baby is likely to be distressed and fretful as a result.

Thrush is easily treated by drops which your doctor will prescribe for you, but don't delay in taking the baby to him. The disorder is infectious, and you should take special care about keeping the baby's bottles, etc. away from the rest of the family crockery. Wash your hands carefully after feeding him.

Vaginal Thrush

This is one of the commonest forms of vaginal discharge, and, though no accurate figures exist, it wouldn't be at all surprising if it transpired that 25% of women have vaginal thrush at some time in their lives. The condition is very frequently encountered in pregnancy, and also in diabetic women.

The discharge that thrush produces is thick and white, and there will be associated soreness, and irritation. The diagnosis is confirmed by a simple microscopic examination of a vaginal swab, and treatment with nystatin (or newer anti-thrush pessaries) is normally curative. It's important, however, to persist with the full course, which may take up to two weeks, depending on the doctor's advice. Recurrences do tend to occur, but can readily be treated in the same way.

Treatment of the partner (or partners) is important too—as is avoiding hot baths and nylon underwear. (The fungus loves warmth and moisture.)

TICS

Tics, or habit spasms, are nearly always of psychological origin, and indicate some underlying stress. If the tic is very trying, specialist help should be sought. But *tic doul-*

oureux is not, in fact, a real tic but an intensely painful form of facial neuralgia. Drugs such as carbamazepine are useful in relieving the condition, but it may be necessary to resort to nerve surgery to 'deaden' the face. (*See also* NEURALGIA.)

TOADSTOOL POISONING

Poisoning by toadstools and other fungi still occurs. It is always wisest to buy mushrooms from a shop rather than picking them yourself, unless you are very experienced and can tell a mushroom from a toadstool with absolute certainty.

The most dangerous fungus is *Amanita phalloides*, the Death Cap, which bears a superficial likeness to the edible mushroom (*Psalliota campestris*). The Death Cap has white gills (as opposed to the brown gills of the edible mushroom), a yellowish top, and a sheath (called a volva) around the base of the stem. Confusion of the two species is very easy.

If you suspect someone has eaten a poisonous fungus, make him vomit and then get him to hospital as fast as possible. Take any vomit matter (and any pieces of fungus that have not been eaten) along with you.

Warning: After eating a poisonous fungus the patient may feel fine for several hours. The initial symptoms of Death Cap poisoning (abdominal pain, vomiting, diarrhoea, thirst and collapse) may not come on for 15 hours.

TOBACCO ADDICTION

Nicotine and alcohol are, of course, the commonest of all addictive drugs. Nicotine can be taken either as snuff or tobacco, and there seems at present to be relatively little risk to health from snuff.

Things are different with tobacco, however. Current research suggests that moderate cigar or pipe smoking is relatively harmless, unless you happen to have a chest or heart trouble. Some Swiss and German scientists have suggested that there is a link between lung cancer and both cigar and pipe smoking, but research elsewhere has not so far borne this out. Probably it depends on how you smoke.

There is no question, however, that cigarette smoking greatly increases one's chances of getting lung cancer, a distressing and often painful illness which is nearly always fatal. Only if you smoke less than about five cigarettes a day can you afford to forget this risk.

Cigarette smoking also increases the chances of getting various unpleasant disorders, such as coronary heart disease, chronic bronchitis, emphysema, duodenal ulcer and a number of other less common conditions. The life expectancy of a smoker is therefore considerably less than that of a non-smoker.

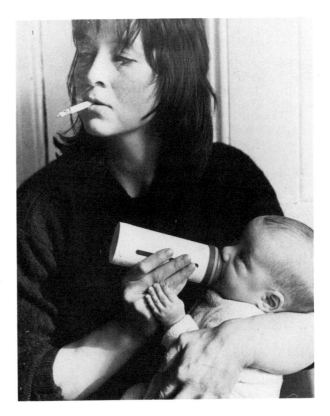

It's encouraging that if a life-long heavy smoker gives up cigarettes altogether, his chances of avoiding lung cancer start to improve shortly afterwards. That's why doctors' lung cancer rates have dropped dramatically in recent years. It's therefore always worth trying to break the habit.

Giving Up Smoking

There is no easy way of giving up smoking, and no magic drug that will break the addiction. A recent survey by the Consumers Association of 'smoking cures' on sale to the public showed that most of them were of little value at all.

The best course is probably to select a particular date, say the following Monday, and decide to give up completely on that day. The next week is likely to be extremely unpleasant, but once you've got through it it's probable that your dependence on nicotine will be broken. Don't be tempted afterwards to have the odd cigarette in moments of stress, or perhaps at a party, or you may well find yourself hooked again.

Giving up smoking, like giving up many other things (such as alcohol or food), is much easier in pairs or groups. It's very hard to backslide when you know that half a dozen other people have heard you undertake to give up completely. Withdrawal symptoms are also easier to bear when you know that your companions are going through the same miseries as yourself. There are a number of 'Anti-Smoking Clinics' which organize group therapy (*see under* **Good Sense About Smoking and Drinking** in the chapter called A GUIDE TO A HEALTHY LIFE).

Incidentally, your doctor may sometimes (though not always) be willing to help you alleviate your withdrawal symptoms by prescribing you a week's course of a mild tranquillizer. This may help you through the difficult period without getting you hooked on the tranquillizing drug instead of nicotine. Some patients are able to give up with the aid of hypnotism, but make sure you select a proper medical hypnotist—that is, a doctor, and not someone who does palm-reading in their spare time!

A new preparation of nicotine chewing gum—Nicorette—does seem to help a lot of people. But you have to be careful not to get hooked on the gum!

If You Can't Give Up

If the addiction is too strong for you to break, try at least to lessen the risk to your health as far as possible.

First, switch from cigarettes to a pipe or cigars (small cigars are quite acceptable for women nowadays!). If you can't give up cigarettes, cut them down. If you're smoking 20 a day try to aim initially for 15, for instance by setting a fixed interval of not less than 45 minutes or so between smokes.

Use a filter-tip and low-tar brand and try to throw cigarettes away when only half or three-quarters smoked. This may be hard on the pocket, but it's better for the health—the last inch or so of the cigarette is the most dangerous part.

Finally, always take the cigarette out of your mouth between puffs. It's been shown that letting it dangle continuously from the lips increases the danger of lung cancer considerably, because you inhale more muck.

TOENAIL, INGROWING

An ingrowing toenail can be very painful indeed. Factors causing it are *(a)* wearing overtight shoes especially in early life; and *(b)* using the wrong method of trimming the nail (see below).

Often, however, an ingrowing toenail just seems to happen with no very obvious cause.

Care of the Toenails

Toenails should always be trimmed straight across and not in a curve. Try not to dig the scissors into the soft flesh at either end. Doctors used to tell patients to cut a 'V' in the middle of the nail, but nowadays this isn't generally considered to be much help. It's also blooming difficult.

It should go without saying that everybody should try and keep their toenails as clean as possible. If you fail to scrub the nails properly, getting the brush into the little crevices on each side, it's all too easy for germs to collect and infection to arise.

Treatment of Ingrowing Toenail

If a toenail does become ingrowing despite careful hygiene, see your doctor who may advise you to have regular foot care from a podiatrist or chiropodist. If things have got too bad, however, he'll arrange for some form of minor surgical procedure on the toe.

Most commonly, surgery just involves having a piece of toenail cut away (quite painlessly, under local anaesthetic). It may be necessary to remove the whole nail, however (don't worry, it'll soon grow again!). And a new operation involves putting a little 'gutter' in alongside the nail.

Sometimes, ingrowing toenail is so troublesome that the surgeon feels it best to remove the whole nail *bed*—that is, the area from which the nail grows. Of course, you will never have a toenail after this operation, but virtually all patients are only too glad to be rid of the nuisance and the pain.

Ingrowing toenail often leads to the development of a whitlow, or run-around (*see under* NAIL DISORDERS). If your toe becomes red, inflamed and sore, or if you notice pus at the side of the nail, then try to see your doctor within the next day or so. Meanwhile, bathe the foot in hot, soapy water every four hours.

TONGUE DISORDERS

There are few serious disorders of the tongue. A lot of people get alarmed by unusual appearances of the tongue, but these are rarely of significance.

True Diseases

LARGE ULCERS OR HARD SORES. These should be seen by a doctor, as soon as possible. They may be trivial in nature, but hard sores particularly could be a symptom of at least two serious diseases, both of which need immediate treatment.

SMALL ULCERS. These can be painful and very trying. Gargling with hot salt water or an application of gentian violet may help to clear them up, but if they persist longer than a few days, see your doctor, who'll probably prescribe a steroid tablet to suck.

SORE, SMOOTH, SHINY TONGUE. This may indicate iron or, more rarely, vitamin deficiency. See your doctor as soon as you can.

Unusual Appearances

FURRED TONGUE: People worry about a furred tongue, but this appearance rarely means anything more than that the patient has been breathing through his mouth overnight. A hangover is another cause, and furring is also seen in many smokers.

When abnormal furring of the tongue occurs because of disease, other symptoms of the illness will usually have occurred well beforehand.

BLACK 'HAIRY' TONGUE. This appearance is sometimes seen when a patient has been taking antibiotics, but often it occurs for no known reason. The condition usually disappears of its own accord.

GEOGRAPHICAL TONGUE. Quite a lot of people have tongues that are covered with lines, giving the appearance of a map. This finding is of no significance.

LARGE PINK SPOTS FAR BACK ON THE TONGUE. People quite often notice these and go to the doctor about them. Usually it turns out that all they are seeing is the taste buds at the back of the tongue.

TONSILS AND TONSILLITIS

The tonsils are a part of the body's defences against infection, and inflammation of the tonsils (tonsillitis) indicates that they are doing their job in trapping and attacking germs inhaled through the mouth and nose.

Occasional episodes of tonsillitis are, therefore, to be expected in childhood. A lot of parents don't appreciate this, and want their children's tonsils removed after only a few bouts. Perhaps this attitude is understandable—after all, a generation or so ago (when most of today's parents were children), doctors too were very keen on tonsillectomy. This isn't so today, however; general practitioners, surgeons and pediatricians are very conscious of the possible dangers of removal of the tonsils. Complications after the operation are quite frequent, and it's often a thoroughly upsetting experience for the child.

So, if your child has had a number of attacks of tonsillitis, please don't try to pressurize your doctor into arranging an operation if he doesn't think it's indicated. If you've discussed it with him and you're still in doubt, you might do well to talk things over with a pediatrician as well.

Acute Tonsillitis

This is one of the commonest of all childhood illnesses. People tend to regard it with rather more seriousness than it deserves, because, after all, it's only the equivalent of a sore throat in an adult, though it can be pretty miserable.

SYMPTOMS. Children (and especially young children) very often don't seem to feel soreness at the back of the throat in the same way as adults do.

It's more likely that a child with tonsillitis will just lose his appetite, develop a raised temperature, and vomit. He may also have a cough, and the glands at the side of his neck are likely to be enlarged.

TREATMENT. Don't try to persuade the child to eat against his will—he'll probably want to vomit the food back. Until the doctor comes, just give him cold drinks and a little aspirin, and keep him as cool as possible, particularly if his temperature is very high. (For methods of keeping the temperature down, *see* TEMPERATURE.) The doctor will give him antibiotics and he'll very likely be better in a few days.

TOOTHACHE

Toothache can vary in intensity from a slightly painful reaction to cold water, lasting for a matter of seconds, to a continuous pain severe enough to prevent sleep at night.

The only way to deal with any form of dental pain is to make an appointment and see your dentist. Home remedies are at best a temporary expedient. In the case of severe pain, take two aspirin (or other similar analgesic tablets) every four hours until you get to see the dental surgeon. Some people place aspirin tablets on the gum beside an aching tooth, but this isn't a good idea because it may cause an unpleasant burn.

If there is swelling (which may be caused by an abscess), or soreness of the gums over the wisdom teeth, keep washing the mouth out with hot saline—*i.e.* a teaspoonful of salt in a glass of hot water.

The time-honoured popular remedy for toothache is oil of cloves. If the aching tooth has a large cavity caused by neglected decay or the loss of a filling, a small piece of cotton wool soaked in oil of cloves can be placed in the hole as a temporary measure only.

Most toothache is quite unnecessary and wouldn't occur if people attended their dentists for regular check-ups at six-month intervals and cleaned their teeth really thoroughly and regularly. It's also a good idea for children to use fluoride toothpaste.

TOXAEMIA OF PREGNANCY (*See under the heading* **Pre-eclampsia** in PREGNANCY.)

TRAVEL SICKNESS

Nausea and vomiting while travelling in a car, plane, or ship, are very common. These symptoms are made worse by psychological factors, such as anxiety. In car- and air-sickness particularly, it's often true that the patient frightens himself into being sick. Once a person develops confidence that he can travel by car or plane without becoming ill, from then on everything's usually all right.

Sea-sickness is in a slightly different category, however. Though psychological factors do play a part (especially in the person who comes on board a ship at the dockside, walks straight over to the rail and is sick!), physical factors are very important. The repetitive motion of the waves produces a disruptive effect on the stomach itself, and on the balancing mechanisms of the inner ear. Many physiologists believe that a sufficiently prolonged up-and-down movement will make anyone (however good a sailor) vomit after a time!

Treatment

The motion sickness remedies on sale to the public are quite effective. They have two separate actions. Firstly, they 'damp down' the balance mechanisms of the ear and, secondly, they reduce anxiety about the possibility of vomiting. Take them only in the dosage recommended, however, and don't use them if you are going to drive a car—this could be very dangerous. (Of course, people who are driving are very rarely travel sick, because their minds are much too occupied with the job in hand.) If the proprietary remedies don't work, consult your doctor.

Car-Sick Children

If you never mention the idea of car-sickness to children, they probably won't ever get sick. If your child does show a tendency this way, try and treat the problem in a matter-of-fact fashion. Don't keep discussing it with him before you start out, or ask him if he feels sick throughout the journey. *Just have a stout paper bag ready, and produce it if necessary.*

The chances of sickness are reduced if you make sure there's plenty of fresh air going through the car, and if you stop every now and again to let the child stretch his legs. In between stops, keep him occupied at all costs—with games, puzzles or stories.

Some people believe that car-sickness is due to static electricity, and hang a chain from the car to let the alleged charge pass into the ground. This might work if you can persuade the children to believe in it, but it doesn't have any scientific basis.

TRICHOMONAS INFECTION OF THE VAGINA

Trichomonas vaginalis (often rather confusingly called 'TV' for short) is a very common cause of vaginal discharge and irritation, particularly during pregnancy or bouts of ill-health. It is caused by a microscopic parasite.

The characteristic feature of trichomonas infection is a profuse yellow discharge, often full of little bubbles. The vulva becomes so sore that intercourse is difficult or impossible.

Treatment is a fairly simple business though recurrences are liable to occur. The doctor can arrange a microscopic examination to confirm the diagnosis and will then prescribe a course of tablets lasting perhaps a week. It's very important to go right through to the end of this course without missing any doses. The patient's husband should also take a course of the tablets at the same time, since otherwise the parasite will continue to be passed to and fro at intercourse. (Trichomonas may be carried by the man, but rarely produces symptoms in him.)

TUBERCULOSIS

An infection caused by a germ called *Mycobacterium tuberculosis*. TB used to be one of the great scourges of mankind. People called it 'the white plague', and if you ever have the chance to look at death certificates of 50 or 60 years ago, you'll see why. Time and again (and particularly among the young) you'll find the cause of death stated as 'Pulmonary (*i.e.* lung) tuberculosis', or (in older certificates) 'Phthisis' or 'Consumption'.

The incidence of TB has fallen dramatically in all Western countries over the last 30 years or so. The great successes which have been achieved are partly due to anti-TB drugs, but also in very large measure to the tremendous work which has been done in the public health field.

Although TB cases (and TB deaths) continue to diminish in number, this is still not a rare disease by any means, and it's essential that we keep up our vigilance against it. For instance, it's important that all schoolchildren should be tested for susceptibility to TB. Most kids *are* susceptible and will need BCG (anti-TB) vaccination.

Pulmonary Tuberculosis

This is TB of the lungs. The germ is spread by the cough of infected persons, and is breathed in through the nose and mouth before lodging in the lungs. Very often the infection comes to nothing, and the patient never realizes that he has had a mild TB infection until an X-ray or skin test reveals the fact, perhaps years later. Thirty years ago, the majority of city children could be shown to have had such an unnoticed infection, but nowadays only a small proportion of children show a positive skin reaction indicating past infection.

TB of the lungs may take a far more serious turn, however, if the disease becomes well-established and isn't overcome by the body's defences. Symptoms of pulmonary TB include: unexplained cough persisting for longer than two weeks; pink or blood-stained sputum; unexplained weight loss; episodes of sweating at night; vague general ill-health.

If you have any of these symptoms, see your doctor, who will examine you and, if necessary, order a chest X-ray.

TB Elsewhere in the Body

Tuberculosis can effect many other organs apart from the lungs—for instance, the intestine, the joints, the neck glands and the kidneys.

Some such infections are acquired in the same way as lung TB, that is, from the cough of an infected person. However, some cases still originate from drinking infected milk, particularly abroad.

People tend to think that milk is always pure and wholesome, but this isn't necessarily so. Ideally, all milk consumed by humans should be pasteurized and should come from cattle which have been shown to be free of TB. This may not be so *(a)* in country districts, and *(b)* when you are on holiday abroad. Don't be tempted to drink raw milk 'fresh from the cow', however healthy the local people think it is. (It regularly gives people other things apart from TB!)

The symptoms of TB outside the lung vary so greatly that it's not practicable to describe them in full here. They include swelling of bones and joints, enlarged neck glands, persistent skin ulceration and recurrent urinary infections.

Treatment

TB, whether in the lungs or elsewhere, can almost always be cured now, provided it is caught early enough. Prolonged stays in a sanitorium are very rarely necessary today, and some patients don't even have to go into hospital. Treatment is usually quite prolonged, however, and most patients are put on drug therapy for a period of a year or so. A combination of drugs is usually given, and the commonest preparations used are streptomycin (which has to be given by injection), PAS, and isoniazid. It's absolutely vital that the drugs are taken regularly and without fail throughout the course. Regular check-ups will be necessary for some years after the patient is cured.

In most advanced countries, public health workers will arrange for chest X-rays and skin tests to be carried out on a new TB patient's family and close contacts. This contact-checking is a very important part of the battle to exterminate the disease. If you're a friend or relative of someone who has TB, it doesn't matter how healthy you think you are or how well you feel—have a check-up right away.

TUMOURS

The word 'tumour' simply means a swelling, which may be either benign or malignant. It does not necessarily imply cancer. Malignant tumours are discussed under the heading CANCER, and also under the names of individual organs.

TWIN PREGNANCY

Twins occur roughly once in every 80 or 90 deliveries. They often run in families. There are two types, identical and non-identical.

Identical twins are formed from one egg (ovum) and one sperm. After the egg has been fertilized by the sperm, it splits in two, and the two halves develop into two separate babies. They will be of the same sex, and indeed identical in every way.

Non-identical twins are formed from two separate eggs, each of which is fertilized by a different sperm. The twins so formed have no more in common than ordinary brothers and sisters would have. They may be of the same or different sexes.

Pregnancy

Without special methods (such as ultrasound) twin pregnancy is unlikely to be diagnosed before the 20th week of pregnancy, and most mothers don't find out they are going to have twins until they are about 26–30 weeks pregnant.

The suspicion of twins is most commonly aroused if an expectant mother's girth seems abnormally large for her dates. A woman who normally has a waist measurement of about 26 inches would normally put on roughly one inch per week after the 26th week—making her about 40 inches round the waist when she's nearly ready to deliver.

So, if you're 28 weeks pregnant and your waist measurement is 34 inches, there ought to be some reason why. It could just be fat, or it could be excess accumulation of fluid in the womb (hydramnios), but it could be twins. Careful examination of your tummy may give your doctor the answer, but he'll need an ultrasound scan to be certain.

Once the diagnosis is made, you'll need a little extra antenatal care from your doctor. There are several problems that are commonly encountered in twin pregnancies, but these can be dealt with provided you take the doctor's advice, particularly with regard to rest.

Toxaemia of pregnancy (*see* **Pre-eclampsia** *under* PREGNANCY) is commoner where a multiple birth is expected. So is anaemia, because the two babies need that much more iron from their mother than one child would. The minor disorders of pregnancy (heartburn, nausea, varicose veins and so on) are sometimes liable to be a bit more troublesome than usual, and of course the mother gets tired very easily with all this weight to carry around.

Because of the great importance of ensuring adequate rest and adequate nutrition, many obstetricians hospitalize all patients expecting twins from about the 30th to about the 36th weeks of pregnancy. This may be irksome for you, but please go along with the doctor's advice.

Labour and Delivery

PREMATURITY. Labour often occurs much earlier than expected. Even if it comes on at the normal time, the babies may still be very small. Any baby of under five-and-a-half pounds (2,640 grammes) birthweight is regarded as premature by definition (and therefore needing special care) regardless of how long he's spent in his mother's womb (*see* PREMATURITY in the A–Z of Emergencies).

OTHER PROBLEMS. You may have heard all sorts of alarming tales of complications occurring during twin delivery. Complications certainly do occur sometimes, but there's no reason why all should not go well provided you have had proper antenatal care and are having the delivery in a well-equipped hospital under the care of an experienced obstetrician. (No matter what part of the world you are in, you should always go into hospital for a twin delivery—home delivery could be very risky indeed.)

MECHANISM OF DELIVERY. How do twins actually get out without becoming jammed? What usually happens is simply that the first baby is born in the normal way. The mother's contractions then cease for a short time while the womb 'rests'. After five or 10 minutes, the contractions return, but it usually takes only four or five good contractions for the mother to push the second baby out.

If contractions don't return, the obstetrician will take prompt steps to stimulate them and to get the baby out. You may have heard stories of mothers lying in labour for days waiting for the birth of their second twin (in 1937, a medical journal reported a case of a 92-day interval between twin deliveries!), but today that doesn't happen.

TYPHOID FEVER

Typhoid and paratyphoid (types A, B and C) together make up the enteric group of fevers. ('Enteric' means relating to the bowel.)

The features of all these diseases are broadly similar, and they are all passed on in exactly the same way. The germs which cause them (members of the Salmonella group) are passed out in the bowel motions of infected people, some of whom may not know that they are carrying the germs. If these germs contaminate someone else's food or drink, infection will probably result.

It's very easy for this to happen in most countries of the world. Only in a relatively small number of developed countries can one be sure that sewage material does not contaminate the drinking water supply. In addition, a typhoid carrier who doesn't wash his hands carefully after having a bowel action can all too easily spread germs onto other people's food, and many outbreaks occur in this way.

Features and Treatment of Typhoid

The incubation period of typhoid is seven to 21 days. The onset of symptoms is usually gradual, with slight fever, general feelings of ill-health, headache and loss of appetite. Within a day or two, there is usually quite severe diarrhoea, which may be bloodstained.

Hospital treatment under isolation is essential. With modern fluid replacement and antibiotic therapy, the chances of survival are good. The main risk to life occurs if treatment has begun too late. When on holiday in a typhoid region, always go to a local doctor as soon as possible if you feel ill.

Warning: You may become a typhoid 'carrier' without having any symptoms whatever. 'Carriers' often feel perfectly healthy for years, even though they are excreting typhoid germs the whole time.

Prevention

If you are going to a typhoid region (and this means most countries of the world, including the popular resort areas of Spain, Mexico and North Africa), go to your doctor for a course of typhoid shots first.

Ideally, you should get the first injection some months in advance, but an abbreviated course starting one month before leaving gives reasonable protection. Unless you have a good travel agent, it's unlikely that he will tell you of the need to get immunized. Unfortunately, the jab is sometimes the most painful one of all!

Once you reach the typhoid area, take care, even if you've been immunized. Drink only boiled or purified water, and beware of unboiled milk.

You can't protect yourself against every source of enteric fever, but it's common sense to avoid eating places that seem dirty and unhygienic. In camping and caravan sites particularly, you should take great care about washing your hands before preparing food and after going to the toilet.

U

ULCERS

An ulcer is a breach in the skin or any of the mucous membranes of the body. Stomach (gastric) and duodenal ulcers are dealt with below, under Peptic Ulcers.

Skin and Mouth Ulcers

SKIN. Any skin ulcer which has persisted for more than a couple of weeks, or which is bleeding or getting bigger, needs to be seen by a doctor as soon as possible. A rodent ulcer is a special type of skin ulcer which commonly occurs on the upper part of the face (*see* RODENT ULCER). Varicose skin ulcers are dealt with under the heading VARICOSE ULCERS. Ulcers on the genital region should be seen by a doctor as soon as possible, and preferably within 24 hours.

MOUTH. As with skin ulcers, any mouth ulcer which has persisted for two weeks, or which is bleeding or getting bigger, should be assessed by a doctor without delay.

Small whitish mouth ulcers are a nuisance but are not often serious. Gargling with hot salt water may help, but, if it doesn't, see your doctor.

Recurrent mouth ulceration may be an indication that something is wrong with the teeth—for instance, a rough jagged edge, or a poor 'bite' between upper and lower jaws. If this is the case, your dentist will be able to put things right. (*See also* TONGUE DISORDERS.)

Peptic Ulcers

This term is applied to stomach (gastric) and duodenal ulcers. (There are one or two other rare types of peptic ulcer, but they needn't concern us here.) The duodenum is the short tube that leads out of the stomach.

SYMPTOMS. The characteristic symptom of an ulcer is recurrent pain in the upper part of the abdomen, usually in the midline. This pain is often relieved by taking food, milk or antacids (alkalis). It's made worse by hunger, and may sometimes be aggravated by worry, lack of rest, and smoking.

Other symptoms include the passing of black, tarry motions (caused by bleeding from the ulcer). Sometimes too, blood may be vomited up (*haematemesis*), and if this happens it will probably have a black 'coffee ground' appearance rather than the natural colour of blood.

It's quite possible to get pain of the ulcer type when you haven't got an ulcer: this symptom is particularly common among people who've been overworking or are under stress in some other way. If you get recurrent upper abdominal pain, however, always see your doctor.

INVESTIGATION. He will examine you and, if he feels you may have an ulcer, he'll order a barium meal X-ray. An ordinary X-ray wouldn't show up an ulcer, so you are given some radio-opaque barium to swallow, and if an ulcer is present this will usually outline it.

You may also have to have blood tests and stool tests (to see if the ulcer is bleeding), and also a special investigation called a gastroscopy in which the specialist inspects the inside of your stomach (or duodenum) with a flexible telescope-like device which is passed through your mouth.

MEDICAL TREATMENT. Most patients with an ulcer are treated medically rather than surgically, at least to begin with.

The first principle of treatment is correct diet. Until quite recently, anyone with an ulcer had to keep to all kinds of dietary restrictions. Some of them were told to avoid all fried and fatty foods, while others lived entirely on milk, rice puddings, and other 'sloppy' dishes.

Nowadays, many doctors feel that it doesn't matter what you eat, as long as you don't let your stomach get empty. 'Little and often' is a good dietary rule. In other words, when you've gone an hour since the last meal, it's time for a snack of, say, a glass of milk and a biscuit.

Smoking is best avoided altogether, and some ulcers cannot be expected ever to heal if the patient goes on smoking.

Rest is important. Try to get eight hours sleep a night. If the pain is bad, and particularly if you have a lot of strain and worry at work, it's often best to take a few days off, spending perhaps the first 24 hours in bed.

Your doctor will prescribe antacid and other drugs which will relieve symptoms, though they do not heal the ulcer. In the 1960s, however, a preparation called carbenoxolone was introduced. This is based on the traditional stomach remedy of liquorice, and it has been shown to heal a high proportion of gastric ulcers. A separate preparation is available for treating duodenal ulcers, but its value as a healing agent hasn't as yet been proven.

Since that time, new British-invented drugs such as Zantac and Tagamet have come in. They're very effective, despite criticism of their possible long-term safety.

SURGICAL TREATMENT. Your doctor may decide that you

should see a surgeon, particularly if you are getting severe symptoms which are not responding to therapy, or if you have run into complications, such as heavy bleeding.

If the surgeon decides to operate, he may carry out one of several procedures. Partial gastrectomy means removal of the major part of the stomach; vagotomy means cutting through the nerves that supply the stomach. Both these procedures are designed to cut down on acid production.

These operations give very good results in the majority of cases, but some people have very troublesome symptoms afterwards, such as persistent diarrhoea, or inability to eat more than very small quantities of food. Not all patients are suitable for operation, anyway, so don't try to pressurize the surgeon to operate on you if he doesn't feel it would be a good idea. Some ulcer patients do this, and are often very disappointed with the results afterwards.

ULCERATIVE COLITIS

This is a trying disorder the characteristic feature of which is gross inflammation of the large intestine (the colon and rectum). Its symptoms include persistent severe diarrhoea, rectal bleeding, weight loss and general ill-health. During attacks, there may be 20 or 30 bowel movements a day.

The cause of ulcerative colitis isn't really known. Many doctors believe that it's caused by the body forming anti-bodies against its own tissues. Some think that psycho-logical factors play a part in causing the disease and point to the fact that many patients with ulcerative colitis are tense and suffer with anxiety; on the other hand, the illness itself is so distressing that it's not really surprising that patients show signs of strain.

Although it may be hard to believe during the early attacks, which can be very severe, the outlook these days is quite good. New drugs are available for treating ulcera-tive colitis, and the anti-inflammatory steroids, given in enema form, have proved of great value.

A minority of patients undergo surgery, usually having the whole of the large intestine removed. This sounds very drastic, but in fact it often produces a wonderful improve-ment, and can revolutionize the person's life.

A very small number of sufferers improve greatly if milk is cut out of their diet.

Anyone with ulcerative colitis should remain under a specialist's care even during long periods of good health. Regular check-ups are essential because of the risk of serious complications.

URINARY DISORDERS (See BED-WETTING, CYSTITIS, PYELITIS and RETENTION OF URINE;

KIDNEYS AND PROSTATE GLAND in the A–Z of Parts of the Body.)

URTICARIA

Urticaria, often known as 'hives' or 'nettle rash', is an allergic skin condition. Affected areas of skin become raised, puffy and reddened. Agents which may provoke attacks include medicines, various kinds of food (especially eggs, shellfish and strawberries) and plants.

Antihistamine drugs are usually of value in treating attacks of urticaria. If the attacks are recurrent, the doctor will try, by careful testing, to identify the agent to which the patient is allergic, but this is not always possible.

V

VD (*See* VENEREAL DISEASES.)

VACCINATION

Vaccination originally meant simply immunization against smallpox (*see* SMALLPOX), but the word is now used to indicate any kind of immunization (*see* IMMUNIZATION in the chapter 'The Seven Ages of Man (and Woman)').

VARICOSE VEINS

These are widened and tortuous veins under the skin of the leg. (Similar varicosities may occur in the rectum, where they are called piles, in the gullet, in the scrotum, and on the vulva.)

Often, it's not clear why a person has developed varicose veins, but obesity and pregnancy are factors which can play an important part. Wearing a tight girdle over a period of years can also increase a tendency to varicosity.

Complications

BLEEDING. Sometimes a varicose vein bursts, particularly after some minor injury to the shin region. The resulting bleeding may be alarming and prompt action is necessary.

Lie the patient down flat, raise his leg well up in the air and keep it there. Apply a clean pad (*e.g.* a freshly laundered handkerchief) over the bleeding point, and bind it in place firmly but not tightly. Keep the patient lying flat and the leg elevated on a pile of cushions till medical help arrives. (*See also* BLEEDING in A–Z of Emergencies.)

VARICOSE ULCERS. These are quite common in patients with long-standing varicose veins. They occur just above the ankle on the inner side of the skin and are often surrounded by an area of eczema. Far and away the most important aspect of treatment is rest, with the ulcer raised well above the level of the heart. Ideally, the patient should lie down with his foot on a pile of cushions for three or four hours a day. The doctor will prescribe a firm bandage and also skin applications, but the latter are of little importance compared with the need for rest.

Treatment of Varicose Veins

IN PREGNANCY. Mild varicosities occurring for the first time during pregnancy may well disappear after the birth of the baby. Draw your doctor's attention to the veins; he will probably prescribe more rest with your feet up on cushions. You might need to wear elastic support tights for the duration of the pregnancy.

AT OTHER TIMES. In obese patients, mild varicose veins may well respond to weight reduction. Elastic support tights or stockings are also helpful. In moderate or severe cases, a complete cure can be achieved by means of surgery. The cosmetic results of removal of varicose veins are very good in skilled hands, and there should only be a few tiny scars on the skin afterwards. *Injection* of varicose veins is a more minor procedure, but the cosmetic results may not be so beautiful.

VASECTOMY

Vasectomy is male sterilization. This is an increasingly popular method of family limitation, and we've now reached the stage where astonishingly large numbers of men have the procedure carried out when they and their wives feel that they have as many children as they want. (A wife's written consent to vasectomy should be, of course, essential.)

Vasectomy is carried out by cutting through the two tubes (one on each side) which carry the sperm upwards from the testicles. It's usually done under local anaesthetic, and the doctor usually makes two very small incisions, one on each side of the scrotum, though it's possible to carry out the operation through one mid-line incision.

There is little pain afterwards, though many patients get some bruising, which usually takes a week to heal.

Sperm tests on the seminal fluid must be carried out afterwards in case the patient is still fertile—many doctors perform this check at about three months after the operation. It's essential for the couple to continue using some form of birth control until the doctor tells them that the test is OK.

Vasectomy appears to have no effect whatever on sexual function. Some patients find that their married life is greatly improved once the risk of unwanted pregnancy is taken away. It's possible, however, that a man who is mentally ill (and particularly someone suffering from castration fears or worries about virility) could run into emotional problems, such as psychological impotence, after the operation. Preferably, such a person should be persuaded against having a vasectomy in the first place.

At the present time, it's best for a couple who are considering a vasectomy to assume that the operation is irreversible. Some surgeons have had a degree of success in reconnecting the tubes, but in general you should only have a vasectomy if you are absolutely certain that you are never going to want to have any more children.

However, in a few years, things may be different. Research is being carried out on a miniature tap which could be implanted in the tube that carries the sperm and turned on or turned off at will!

Suggestions, based on work with a small number of monkeys, that vasectomy might provoke artery disease have not yet been borne out.

VENEREAL DISEASES

VD is common nowadays, particularly among teenagers. Not enough people realize this fact, which is one reason why these diseases keep on spreading. Anyone who has had a casual sexual liaison would be well advised to go to a hospital 'Special Clinic' for a check-up, *under conditions of strict anonymity.* A few simple tests carried out there will tell whether infection has taken place. (These clinics are advertised quite widely nowadays. If in doubt, ring the nearest large hospital and enquire when the next 'Special Clinic' will be held, or call the Family Planning Information Service at 01-636 7866.)

It's important to bear in mind that VD in women (and occasionally in men) may well produce no obvious symptoms. Therefore, if you have the least suspicion of it, have a check at once. Treatment, if carried out right away, is usually curative.

Prevention

VD is virtually always passed on by having sexual contact (though not necessarily actual intercourse) with an infected person. Repeated contact is not necessary—a few seconds will suffice.

It's obvious, therefore, that VD would be rapidly wiped out in a world in which everybody was always faithful to his or her sexual partner. Blatant promiscuity, or 'sleeping around', is very likely to lead to infection, particularly in cities, large towns, and ports, where the incidence of VD is always high. Unfortunately, 'new' infections like herpes are beginning to spread alarmingly in such areas.

In Britain, and some other countries, it's been shown statistically that a man who goes with street prostitutes is virtually certain to get VD before long.

Wearing a sheath and washing carefully immediately after intercourse provides at least some protection against venereal infection, but not much; it's far more sensible to avoid 'sleeping around'.

If you suspect that infection has occurred, cease all sexual activity at once in case you spread the disease further. If the clinic find that you actually *do* have VD, you'll probably be given tracing slips to give to anyone you've slept with recently. Though it's embarrassing, always pass these on: otherwise the consequences for these people (and their future sexual contacts) may be disastrous.

(*See also* GONORRHEA, NON-SPECIFIC URETHRITIS, AND SYPHILIS.)

VERRUCA

This word just means a wart (*see* WARTS) on the sole of the foot. For some reason, girls' schools tend to get in a bit of a state about verrucas, and children who have them are sometimes treated almost as if they were lepers. This is quite unnecessary—it's a trivial condition that usually responds fairly quickly to treatment by a chiropodist—current cost: about £3–£4 a visit. Doctors will prescribe anti-verruca gels, but these are less certain in their effects. Unless the doctor specifically advises against it, there's no need to give up sports, though shoes should be worn while using the changing room, and a rubber 'verruca sock' in pools and showers.

VERTIGO

A sensation in which the surroundings seem to spin around one, either from right to left or vice versa. It's usually accompanied by nausea and vomiting, and sometimes by noises in the ears.

Vertigo is much less common than ordinary dizziness (*see* DIZZINESS), and is of much more importance. It usually indicates some disorder of the balance mechanisms of the inner ear, such as Menière's disease (*see* MENIÈRE'S DISEASE.)

If you get an attack of true vertigo, as opposed to dizziness, always see your doctor about it as soon as possible. Once the diagnosis is made, the condition can often be helped by anti-vertigo drugs.

VITAMIN DEFICIENCY

Vitamin deficiency is almost unknown these days among adults living in temperate climates. If you want to spend money on expensive vitamin pills, you probably won't do yourself any harm, but you won't do yourself any good either. It's best to show the formula on the bottle to your doctor first, just in case there's anything there that might not be good for you.

Old people occasionally need supplements of vitamin C, particularly where they don't get much in the way of fruit and vegetables, but they are best prescribed by a doctor.

Women in early pregnancy—and women who are trying to get pregnant—may need folic acid supplements.

Children

Babies and young children are often given supplements of vitamins A, D and C. A and D are usually given together, usually in the form of fish liver oils. Vitamin C is given in specially prepared orange or tomato juice, or as rose-hip syrup. Vitamin D is important for Asian children living in cities where there isn't a lot of sunlight.

Women on the Pill

Women who are depressed on the Pill—and also women with premenstrual tension—sometimes seem to benefit from vitamin B6 (pyridoxine).

VOMITING

The causes of vomiting usually lie either within the abdomen or within the skull ('central' vomiting). The former is much more common.

Abdominal Causes

The most frequently-encountered causes of vomiting are 'stomach upsets' (*see* GASTRITIS AND GASTRO-ENTERITIS). Also common is sickness ('morning sickness') during pregnancy—this can, in fact, occur at any time of day (*see* PREGNANCY). In children, the commonest cause of vomiting is probably acute tonsilitis (*see* TONSILS AND TONSILLITIS), though gastritis and gastro-enteritis are also frequently encountered, as is alcoholism.

Rather less common causes include appendicitis, intestinal obstruction, and bleeding ulcers (*see below*).

'Central' Vomiting

This is very frequently psychological in origin, or at least partly so. Most people have felt sick with apprehension at some time (for instance, before an exam or a job interview). In quite a lot of patients, all kinds of emotional tensions and upsets are expressed as vomiting.

Other 'central' causes include disorders of the inner ear, such as Menière's disease (*see* MENIÈRE'S DISEASE); in such cases, there is usually associated vertigo (*see* VERTIGO). Travel sickness (*see* TRAVEL SICKNESS) also falls into this group, as does the vomiting which so often accompanies migraine attacks (*see* MIGRAINE).

Vomiting of Black or Blood-Stained Material

Black 'coffee-ground' vomit indicates bleeding in or near the stomach. This may be due to ulcers (*see* ULCERS) or other causes, and can be a serious symptom. Lie the patient down. Keep him flat, and call an ambulance. Save any vomited material for inspection.

Bright red blood rarely comes from the stomach, and may actually have been coughed up from the lungs, and not really vomited at all. People quite often mistake bright red medicine for blood. In any case, lie the person down and ring the doctor for advice.

W

WARTS

Warts are small benign growths, caused by a virus. They're commonest on the fingers, wrists, legs and feet, and also the genital areas. They mainly occur in childhood and the teen-age years, and usually disappear by about the age of 25. A lot of doctors think that this is because we develop anti-bodies to the viruses involved.

Whatever their cause, almost all warts will go away in the end. (That is why 'wart charming' so often works!) If a boy or girl has a small wart somewhere where it's not causing any trouble, it's usually better to leave it alone.

However, girls in particular often want warts removed, usually for cosmetic reasons though sometimes because of discomfort. The doctor can either prescribe an application to try to burn the wart away, or else cut it out under local anaesthetic. The latter procedure will probably cause a little pain, but is more likely to lead to cure.

Warts on the penis or vulva should definitely be removed —usually by careful applications of a special paint. (*See also* VERRUCA.)

WAX IN THE EARS

Most people produce a small amount of ear wax but some of us manufacture a great deal. In late middle and old age, wax may make a patient temporarily deaf, especially if water gets behind the 'wall' of wax in the ear (for instance, while swimming). Simple syringing of the ears by the doctor will restore the hearing to normal.

Ear drops that dissolve wax can be bought over the counter, but these aren't a great deal of use when the ear is already blocked. On the other hand, people who get a lot of wax can profitably use these drugs, say, once a week to keep blockage from occurring. Oddly enough, the Pill reduces your chance of getting ear wax trouble.

WHITLOW (*See* NAIL DISORDERS.)

WHOOPING COUGH

Pertussis (as it's known medically) is a common infection, caused by a germ called *Bordetella pertussis*.

It's not such a trivial disease as people often imagine. Though it usually does little harm to adults and older child-ren, it may be a killer in babies, particularly in the first year of life.

Fortunately, the whooping cough death rate has fallen greatly in the last 30 years or so. Even so, complications such as pneumonia, chronic chest and ear trouble remain fairly common, so the disease has to be treated with respect.

The incidence of whooping cough has increased a lot in the last few years (though actual deaths have remained low)—undoubtedly because of parents' fear of brain damage from the vaccine.

If you're doubtful about letting your youngster have it, then talk things over with your GP and the Child Health Clinic. But if you decide against it, *don't* let your children miss out on the other immunizations!

Features of whooping cough

The incubation period is about 12 days. At the beginning of the illness, the child usually has no more than a cold and a cough, and it's virtually impossible to make the diagnosis at this stage.

After some days (perhaps seven or 10) the cough starts coming in violent bouts. Then the characteristic whoop develops. This isn't part of the cough, but a loud crowing noise as the breath is sucked in after a long paroxysm of coughing. The whooping and coughing may go on for two weeks, and sometimes much longer. Vomiting after cough-ing may be troublesome during this time. Unfortunately, antibiotics are of limited value. Latest research appears to indicate that steroid (cortisone-like) drugs help in severe cases, but not all doctors agree on this.

In addition to the treatment given by the doctor, try to keep your child in as moist an atmosphere as possible. When he's having a bad bout in the middle of the night, he will get a lot of relief if you take him into the kitchen and keep a kettle boiling near him for half an hour or so. If you have an electric kettle, or an old-fashioned steam kettle, you can of course use these in the bedroom. It may be helpful to make a 'tent' of sheets over the child's head and direct the steam into it, but you must, of course, be careful not to scald him with the steam.

You may find it easier to feed him when he's just finished a bout of coughing, whooping and vomiting, because he probably won't have another bout for a little while.

The quarantine period for whooping cough is often stated to be 28 days from the onset of symptoms, but in practice it varies from case to case, and may be much longer for some children. Your doctor will advise on this point.

After care

After recovery from whooping cough, there's no need to molly-coddle your child. On the other hand, bear it in mind the risk of chest complications (*see* BRONCHIECTASIS). If, a few weeks or even a few months later, he doesn't seem to be 'picking up' or keeps getting coughs, take him back to the doctor, who will examine him and probably arrange a chest X-ray.

WIND

People use this term either to mean belching or gas (often referred to as flatus or flatulence) passed from the rectum. The production of a certain amount of flatus each day is perfectly normal. Anxiety may increase the volume of gas, and so may eating certain foods. The popular observation that eating beans leads to 'wind' was confirmed scientifically in 1972. Drinking a good deal of water and eating charcoal biscuits are both said to diminish gas formation. The F-Plan Diet definitely increases it.

If it seems that the amount passed is excessive or unduly offensive, it's best to check with your doctor.

WORMS

There are dozens of kinds of parasitic worms throughout the world, but most of them are fortunately rare in temperate countries. Worms tend to occur mainly in children. Symptoms which may suggest infestation include: severe itching around the anus, unexplained ill health and anaemia, and occasionally abdominal pain. The first sign may be the actual passage of a worm in the stool.

The diagnosis of worms tends to put everybody in a great state of alarm or shame, but it's important to stress that these parasites can attack anybody. Medical treatment is quick and easy, but should be given to the whole family, since it's very likely that some of them are infected too.

After treatment, the doctor will probably want to send a stool specimen or rectal swab to the lab to ensure that the infestation has been cleared up. Fortunately, it's most unlikely that there will be any long-term consequences to the person's health from the sort of worm infestation encountered in cool climates.

Prevention

Train your children to keep their nails clean and trimmed, and not to apply them to their behinds, even if they feel an itch. Get them to wash their hands after going to the toilet and before meals.

De-worm any cats or dogs in the house regularly, and keep them away from food and plates.

In warm climates, don't let children run barefoot on soil, particularly if this may be contaminated with faeces.

WRIST INJURIES

The wrist is very commonly either sprained (*see* SPRAINS) or broken. If you've injured your wrist, and especially if you've fallen on an outstretched hand and feel pain in the area afterwards, always see a doctor and have an X-ray. It's very easy for a fracture of one of the small bones of the wrist to be ignored due to the fact it's causing relatively little pain. But such fractures can have *very* serious consequences if they're neglected.

Ordinary sprains are just treated with a cold compress, a bandage, and often a sling for a day or two.

WRY NECK

This is a disorder in which the head and neck become twisted to one side. Sometimes the patient wakes up in the morning to find himself stuck in this odd position.

Wry neck may be caused by muscle spasm or associated with throat infections. A few cases are due to a structural abnormality of the neck bones and an X-ray may sometimes be a good idea. Psychological factors may play a part, and hysteria (*see* HYSTERIA) sometimes presents itself in this rather bizarre way.

If one of your family suddenly develops a twisted and painful neck, keep him lying flat and get him to hold a moderately warm hot water bottle on the side of the neck toward which the head is turned. Give him some aspirin, and leave him in peace for an hour or so. If he hasn't improved at the end of this time, contact your doctor.

B

BEE STINGS (*See* STINGS.)

BIRTH (*See* LABOUR). Management of emergency child-birth is described under PREMATURITY, since most unexpected deliveries at home tend to be premature ones.

BITES (*See* SNAKE BITE and INSECT BITES in the A–Z of Conditions and *see* DOG BITES in this chapter.)

BLEEDING
First Aid in life-threatening (torrential) haemorrhage.
(Haemorrhage just means bleeding.)

Firm pressure applied for long enough will stop almost any bleeding, however severe.

You have only seconds in which to act. Find a piece of cloth (*e.g.* a hankie, a shirt, a blouse, or the sleeve of a pullover). There is no time to worry about the sterility of the material. Jam it firmly over the jet of blood and hold it there till trained help arrives. Do not peek under the pad to see how you are getting on; maintain continuous pressure. If blood wells or spurts round or through the cloth, press another larger pad down on top.

Do *not* use a tourniquet and do *not* try to control the bleeding by means of 'pressure points' far removed from the site of haemorrhage. Tourniquets are dangerous, and pressure points hard to find.

First Aid in Severe Bleeding
When the haemorrhage is not life-threatening, you have slightly more time. Though you shouldn't delay, you can take a few seconds to select a dressing that is clean, if not necessarily sterile. One from a first aid kit is ideal, but a freshly laundered hankie will do in an emergency. Maintain pressure as above till skilled help arrives.

It is sometimes possible to press the edges of a wound together with the fingers and thus stop the bleeding. The advantage of this method is that you touch only the skin, not the wound itself.

First Aid in Moderate or Trivial Bleeding
Such bleeding will not require medical aid.

Find the cleanest dressing readily available, and proceed as described under the heading ABRASIONS in the A–Z of Conditions.

BREATH-HOLDING ATTACKS
Some small children respond to emotional stress not by having tantrums but by simply gritting their teeth and refusing to breathe. After a minute or so, they become blue in the face and may even lose consciousness; at this stage, normal breathing returns.

This symptom is very alarming for the parents, but they should not seek to startle the child out of his attack by slapping him or splashing him with water. Difficult though it may be to manage, an attitude of calmness and sympathy will give the best results. All children who suffer from breath-holding attacks grow out of them with time.

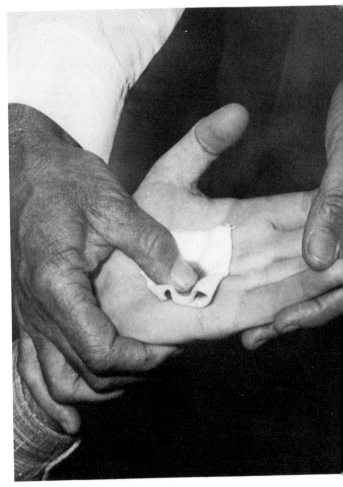

When trying to stop severe bleeding, place a clean dressing directly over the wound and press hard until the flow stops.

BURNS
First Aid

Drench the skin with cold water or any other bland fluid immediately, as in the first few seconds it is most important to reduce the heat of the skin. Take off all *smouldering* clothes very quickly (but carefully so as not to tear off any material stuck to the skin), since they retain heat and will burn the patient further. Once clothes are cool, *don't* try to remove them, as you may cause injury.

If the burns appear severe, lie the victim down, reassure him, and call an ambulance. Resist the temptation to put anything whatsoever on the burned skin, however firmly you or anybody else believes in its healing powers. Do not prick blisters. Remove any *constricting* garments, rings or bangles, since these will cut into burned flesh as it swells.

While waiting for an ambulance, keep the patient comfortable and protected from the cold as he is likely to be suffering from shock (*see* SHOCK in the A–Z of Conditions). If the wait is to be long and there is a risk that the burned area may get infected, use a clean sheet to give protection against germs. Give the patient no solid food, but only sips of water by mouth.

In the case of very *small* burns, pain may safely be relieved with sprays called Burn-Eze, Wasp-Eze or PR Spray, obtainable from a chemist without prescription.

C

CARBON MONOXIDE POISONING (*See* GAS POISONING.)

CHOKING

If a person is choking on something stuck in the top of his/her windpipe, then death can come very swiftly—especially in the case of a child. I've had one of my kids very nearly choke to death on a toy roof tile, and I just managed to 'de-bung' him in time.

In the case of a young child—that is, one who can be lifted—turn him upside down, and smack him sharply several times with the flat of your hand between the shoulder blades.

If this fails, as a 'last-ditch' resort you can stick your forefinger down the child's throat and try to hook out the obstruction. (This worked in my son's case.)

Larger children and adults quite often choke on food—

particularly big pieces of meat. Slap the sufferer hard several times between the shoulder blades to try to dislodge the obstruction.

As an alternative, larger children and adults can be treated by a first-aid technique called 'Heimlich's manoeuvre'. Immediately you realise the person is choking, get behind him and put your arms round his middle. Grasp your own wrist *firmly*, a few inches above his waist.

Now jerk your hands violently inwards and upwards, up to four times. The extreme internal pressure which this produces should blast the obstruction out of his throat.

COMA (For a patient in coma, *see* UNCONSCIOUSNESS).

CONCUSSION (*See* **Brain Injuries** under the heading BRAIN in the A–Z of Parts of the Body.)

CONVULSIONS

Convulsions, or fits may be a manifestation of epilepsy (*see* EPILEPSY in A–Z of Conditions). When they occur for the first time in middle or later life, they may be a symptom of some form of disorder within the brain—for instance, a stroke or a growth (either benign or malignant). These possibilities should be carefully investigated.

Convulsions in childhood are extremely common and are usually due to a high temperature. It used to be thought that they were provoked by teething, but this does not seem likely now. The reason why high temperature so often provokes a fit is that the brain of a baby or toddler is very immature, and often cannot cope with temperatures above about 102°F (38.9°C). When that sort of level is reached, the brain responds with a 'storm' of electrical activity which causes a convulsion.

Vast numbers of children have these 'febrile' (feverish) convulsions, but most of them grow out of them by about the age of five. The immediate first aid treatment is to lower the child's temperature—as described under the heading TEMPERATURE in the A–Z of Conditions. (*See also* EPILEPTIC DISORDERS in the A–Z of Conditions.)

CORONARY THROMBOSIS (HEART ATTACK)

For symptoms, see under the same heading in the A–Z of Conditions. If the patient is conscious, just keep him still and lying flat until a doctor or ambulance arrives.

If breathing or heartbeat have stopped, use the 'kiss of life' and cardiac massage, as described under FIRST AID TECHNIQUES OF RESUSCITATION.

CUTS (*See* BLEEDING)

D

DOG BITES

In a very few countries with strict animal quarantine laws (such as Britain and Eire), dog bites at present carry no more hazard than ordinary cuts or abrasions (*see* ABRASIONS).

Throughout most of the world, however, including much of Europe, excepting the British Isles, any dog must be regarded as a possible source of rabies (*hydrophobia*). Even though the dog may appear perfectly healthy, it is

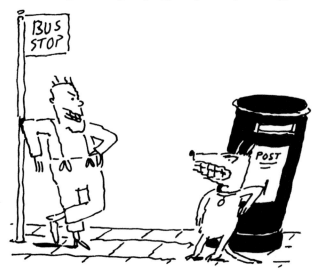

absolutely essential to go straight to a doctor or hospital for anti-rabies vaccination. Once the disease develops it is almost always fatal, so *insist* on the jab, even if people try to fob you off! (This happens, I'm afraid.)

In many parts of the world, wild animal bites are also dangerous. It is best to seek local medical opinion at once if such a bite occurs.

DROWNING

Patients who are apparently drowned can often be saved if prompt action is taken. Get the victim out of the water as fast as possible. If you are on a sloping beach, lie him down on his back so that his head is lower than his feet. Use your finger to clear his mouth of seaweed, vomit or other obstruction. Extract any false teeth. Then give mouth-to-

mouth respiration (the 'kiss of life') as described under the heading FIRST AID TECHNIQUES OF RESUSCITATION. If the heart has actually stopped, the victim needs cardiac massage (also described under FIRST AID) as well, but another person will usually have to carry this out, since it is very difficult for one untrained individual to give both the 'kiss of life' and cardiac massage at the same time.

Keep trying to resuscitate the patient till medical help arrives. Sometimes artificial respiration may have to be continued for as long as a couple of hours before the victim starts breathing on his own.

E

ECLAMPSIA (*See* **Disorders of Pregnancy** under PREGNANCY in the A–Z of Conditions.)

ELECTRIC SHOCK
Domestic Accidents

Severe electric shock can be fatal to the rescuer as well as the initial victim—so be careful. Always switch the current off before you do anything. If this is not possible, stand on some insulating material (*e.g.* rubber or wood) before using a piece of wood (or a rolled-up newspaper, or rubber gloves) to drag or push the patient away from the source of the current.

Next, check that the patient is breathing and that his heart is beating. If necessary, give the 'kiss of life' and cardiac massage (*see under* FIRST AID TECHNIQUES OF RESUSCITATION).

Remember that skin burns from electric shock often turn out to be much worse than they look. Even if such burns seem trivial, take the patient to a hospital or a doctor.

Overhead Cables

The voltages carried in overhead power cables are *very* high indeed. If the victim is thrown clear of the cable, he will probably need immediate resuscitation by means of the 'kiss of life' and cardiac massage (see under FIRST AID TECHNIQUES OF RESUSCITATION). If, however, he is still in contact with the cable, or very near it, do not try to rescue him. Official advice is that nothing can be done until it is certain that the cable has been taken out of service. Even a broken cable lying on the ground near the patient

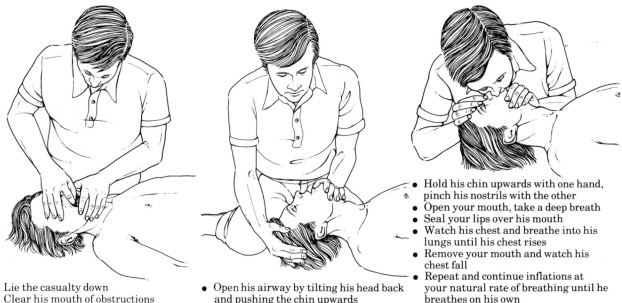

- Hold his chin upwards with one hand, pinch his nostrils with the other
- Open your mouth, take a deep breath
- Seal your lips over his mouth
- Watch his chest and breathe into his lungs until his chest rises
- Remove your mouth and watch his chest fall
- Repeat and continue inflations at your natural rate of breathing until he breathes on his own

- Lie the casualty down
- Clear his mouth of obstructions

- Open his airway by tilting his head back and pushing the chin upwards

may suddenly re-energize. Remember that the current can jump so far that rubber or wood insulating material offers no protection at all.

Therefore, the only course is to keep bystanders about 30 yards back, send someone to contact the police, and wait for official notification that the current has been cut off before moving in to give artificial respiration and cardiac massage.

F

FAINTING (*See* UNCONSCIOUSNESS.)

FIRST AID TECHNIQUES OF RESUSCITATION: THE 'KISS OF LIFE' AND HEART MASSAGE

There are two really vital techniques for use in resuscitation in dire emergency. These are the 'kiss of life' and cardiac massage.

The 'Kiss of Life'

The 'kiss of life' is the most efficient form of artificial respiration but must only be carried out when breathing has stopped. If it is to be done successfully, the patient must have an open airway to allow air to reach his lungs. This is achieved by first clearing the mouth of all debris including vomited material, false teeth etc. Secondly, with the patient lying flat on his back, support the nape of his neck with one hand and press his head backwards with the other until the top of the skull is resting on the ground. Then pull the jaw to keep the mouth open. Unless these procedures are carried out correctly, the tongue will fall back and block the airway, choking the patient to death.

Now open your own mouth wide, take a deep breath, and seal your lips round the patient's mouth. Close off his nostrils with your fingers and then breathe out smoothly and steadily but not hard. Your air will pass into his lungs and his chest should rise. Take your mouth away and wait for a second or two as the air is expelled naturally. Continue this process at a rate of about 20 inflations per minute.

In the case of a baby or young child, seal your lips around the mouth and the nose as well. It is important to blow very, very gently. For a baby, the amount of air you can hold in your cheeks alone should be enough.

Cardiac Massage.

Cardiac massage, or heart massage, can be carried out by a skilled first aider at the same time as the 'kiss of life'. It is very much easier if two people are present, since one can give the 'kiss of life' while the other massages the heart.

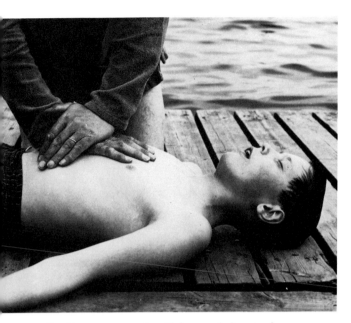

Cardiac massage should be carried out whenever you cannot feel an unconscious person's pulse or heartbeat. Seconds are vital. Lay the patient on a firm surface, such as the floor—a bed does not give sufficient resistance. Place the heel of your hand over the lower part of the breastbone, with the other hand on top. Then rock forward with straight arms so that you press the breastbone down very firmly and smartly—the action should be fairly vigorous. Repeat this pressure once every second. If it is effective, it will produce a pulse which another first aider should be able to feel in the neck or at the wrist. Keep going till the heart restarts.

FITS (*See* CONVULSIONS, and EPILEPSY, in the A–Z of Conditions.)

FRACTURES

(A fracture is the same thing as a break.) Unless you can feel or see the broken end of a bone, it is not possible to tell with any certainty whether a fracture has occurred unless an X-ray is taken. Many people don't realize this and confidently assure their GPs that 'it's not broken, Doctor'. They're then surprised to be sent for an X-ray! If you sustain a severe blow to a bone, with a good deal of pain, it's best to go directly to the nearest hospital Accident Department. Meanwhile the pain can safely be relieved with PR Spray which many sports clubs, etc. have in the first aid kit, or with gentle application of ice.

First Aid

If you suspect someone may have a fracture and you are many miles from medical aid, try to improvise a splint or sling to immobilise and rest the affected arm or leg. To apply a splint efficiently, you really need practical first aid training, but the basic principles are *(i)* to try to immobilize the joints above and below the suspected fracture; *(ii)* to use a really firm splint, *e.g.* a piece of wood or a walking stick; *(iii)* to use thick lashings (*e.g.* handkerchiefs rather than cords) so that they will not cut into the skin; *(iv)* to pad the splint as far as possible. Above all, do not tie the lashings over-tightly, since there is great danger of constricting the circulation and causing gangrene.

Types of Fracture

A *compound* fracture is one in which the skin is broken, allowing germs to enter. It is not (as people often think) one in which the bone breaks into several pieces—this is called a *comminuted* fracture. A *greenstick* fracture is one in which the bone splits longtitudinally, rather than breaking across, as it is bent out of shape; this condition is common in young children. A *complicated* fracture is one in which the broken bone ends damage other structures—nerves, arteries, veins, etc. A *simple* fracture is the ordinary type in which no such complications arise.

If all goes well, the average simple fracture is likely to take about six weeks to mend, but many factors may effect the rate of healing.

GAS POISONING

This used to be caused by the old household gas, but it is now much more often caused by the exhaust fumes from a car engine running in a confined space, or because of the use of a heater in an unventilated place, such as a caravan. If you find a person unconscious in a gas-filled room or a garage or a caravan you must act fast.

Go back into 'clean' air for a few seconds, take several deep breaths and then, holding your breath, dash in and drag the victim outside. If you can turn off the gas (or, in the case of a car, switch off the engine) and throw a window open, so much the better, *but do not risk your life by staying long enough to have to take a breath in the poisonous atmosphere.*

Once you have got the victim out, give him the 'kiss of life' right away (as described under FIRST AID TECHNIQUES OF RESUSCITATION) and keep it up till he starts breathing, or until skilled help arrives. Cardiac massage (described under the same heading) may also be needed.

H

HEAD INJURIES

Head injuries are potentially dangerous and may kill, even when the patient seems perfectly well after the blow. For instance, a young man may be knocked out or slightly dazed while playing football. Unwilling to appear a cissy, he plays on and does not even go to hospital after the match. That night he goes to bed apparently healthy, but is found dead the next morning. Lives are regularly lost because people don't take head injuries seriously enough.

The subject of brain injuries is dealt with more fully under the heading BRAIN in the A–Z of Parts of the Body.

First Aid in Head Injury

Lie the patient down, and keep him flat until he can be taken to hospital for examination and X-ray. Do not leave him alone. If he becomes unconscious, turn him on his side and make sure his mouth is not blocked by vomit, etc. Remove any false teeth.

If breathing stops, give the 'kiss of life', and if the heart stops give cardiac massage. Both these techniques are described under the heading FIRST AID TECHNIQUES OF RESUSCITATION.

I

INJURIES (*See* BLEEDING, BURNS, ELECTRIC SHOCK, FRACTURES, and HEAD INJURIES; DISLOCATIONS and SPRAINS in the A–Z of Conditions.)

L

LABOUR (*Note*: for full details of how to conduct an emergency delivery, see PREMATURITY.)

Although uncomplicated labour is not of course an emergency, it's described here—just in case you go into labour at home and can't get help. It's usual to divide the process of labour into several stages.

The First Stage

The first stage of labour begins with the onset of regular contraction pains, usually with a 'show' (or slight discharge of pink-stained jelly-like material), and sometimes with the 'waters breaking'.

The first stage lasts until the cervix (or neck of the womb) has widened to its maximum, so that the baby's head can pass through it. In a first labour, this stage averages about 10–14 hours, but for a woman who has given birth before, things are usually much quicker—sometimes just an hour.

The Second Stage

The second stage starts at the time when the cervix is widened to its fullest (at which point the mother normally feels a desire to push or 'bear down'). It ends when the baby is born. This takes about an hour or so with a first baby, but again things are often quicker with subsequent children.

The Third Stage

This lasts from the birth of the baby up until when the placenta (afterbirth) has been delivered. No pains are usually felt during this stage, except for the relatively slight contractions which come just before the placenta is expelled.

The 'Fourth Stage'

Although labour is really over once the placenta is out, midwives often use the term 'the fourth stage' to describe the period of weeks before the mother is fully recovered. The idea of this is to stress the fact that she is still far more vulnerable than the average person to all sorts of disorders, including haemorrhage, infection and thrombosis. During this time, therefore, she still needs regular medical or nursing care, followed by advice from the health visitor.

Full details of how to conduct an emergency delivery are given under the heading PREMATURITY—because most emergency births *are* premature ones.

P

POISONING

Treat any case of poisoning as potentially fatal. Never wait to 'see how things go' just because the patient seems quite well, or because you think he hasn't taken very much. Always take the poison or the empty container to hospital with you; if the patient has vomited, take a specimen of the vomited material as well.

First Aid

THE UNCONSCIOUS PATIENT. Turn him on his side, and remove false teeth or anything else (vomit, etc.) blocking the mouth. Make sure he can breathe, as described in the section further on on the care of the unconscious patient under UNCONSCIOUSNESS.

Then phone for an ambulance. Delay in getting the patient to hospital may be fatal.

THE CONSCIOUS PATIENT. If the patient has swallowed a corrosive poison (*i.e.* an acid or alkali), or a petroleum product, do not make him vomit. (If he is screaming in pain, this probably indicates that he has swallowed a corrosive.) Dilute the poison by giving him water to drink. If his mouth or face have been burned by the corrosive, splash water liberally across the skin to wash all traces of it away. Then lie him down and phone for an ambulance.

Most poisons (including all medicinal pills and tablets) are *not* corrosive. Here the first thing to do is to encourage the conscious patient to vomit, either by poking fingers down his throat, or, if this fails, by giving a drink of mustard in water. Then get him to hospital as fast as possible. (If he is still conscious and free from pain, there is no reason why you should not use an ordinary car rather than an ambulance to save time.)

Note: don't waste time searching for antidotes. These seldom exist outside the pages of fiction (and somewhat elderly fiction at that). But take a sample of any likely poison or vomited material with you.

PREMATURITY

A 'prem' is, unfortunately, always at some risk—and a prem delivery outside a hospital is an emergency. By definition, a premature baby is one that weighs less than five and a half pounds (2,640 grammes) at birth. It's possible for a full-time nine-month baby to be premature by this definition, but this is not all that common. Most 'prems' are of eight months gestation or less. A few may have been only five and a half months in the womb, but even today survival rates among these tiny babies of two pounds weight or so are not good.

Among the causes of prematurity are pre-eclamptic toxaemia (*see under* PREGNANCY in the A–Z of Conditions). Vaginal bleeding during the second half of pregnancy may also lead to premature delivery. Twins, triplets, quads and so on are also very likely to be 'prems', as are babies of heavy-smoker mums. In about 50% of cases, however, no cause of prematurity is known.

Emergency Care

There is no need to discuss the *standard* care of the premature baby here, since this is the responsibility of the doctor. If you should have to cope with a 'prem' when far from medical aid, however, remember that the most vital thing is to keep the baby warm at all costs.

The method of delivery is described below. The delivery room should if possible be at a temperature of at least 75°F (24°C) and the child should be received in to a warm thick towel as soon as he is born and make sure his head keeps warm as that's where most heat is lost. *Don't* bathe him, as this will cause a dangerous loss of heat. Once he is breathing, simply wrap the towel around him and tuck him up in a cot under warm blankets. (Don't use a hot water bottle, which may well burn him.) If no cot is available, use a wooden box or a drawer.

How to Carry Out an Emergency Delivery

Fortunately, it's only occasionally that a woman unexpectedly goes into labour when far from medical aid. If you have to cope with such a situation, *keep calm* and don't get flustered. You usually have time to arrange things.

First, try to find time to read briefly through the section on LABOUR (above) and through the remarks above on the emergency care of the premature baby (it's best to assume that an unexpected baby is going to be premature, and take precautions accordingly).

Next, make sure the mother is comfortable in as private a place as you can manage. If no bed is available, spread a sheet of clean plastic (or some newspapers) on cushions or blankets. Reassure her, and keep people away from her. Get some sort of cot or box and plenty of warm towels and blankets ready for the baby as described above.

Ask somebody to find a large quantity of cotton wool, and to boil up lots of hot water and prepare clean jugs and basins. Before the baby is born, scrub your hands and nails thoroughly in a basin of hot water. Let your hands dry in the air—don't use a towel. If they get dirty, scrub them again. Lack of cleanliness on your part may put the lives of mother and child at risk. If you can improvise a mask for yourself (*e.g.* from a clean handkerchief) this will cut down on the chance of your spreading germs to them as well.

THE SECOND STAGE. When the mother reaches the second stage of labour (*see* LABOUR above), she will feel a desire to 'bear down'. Then (and not before), encourage her to push with her pains, but not in the pain-free intervals. When pushing, she can be on her back, with her knees drawn up—or in any other position that's comfortable for her.

THE BIRTH. When a bulge appears at the opening of the vagina, tell the mother to stop pushing. Turn her on her left side with her knees drawn up and her buttocks pushed out towards you at the side of the bed. There are other positions, but they're probably best not attempted by an amateur.

Wash the skin around the vaginal opening with cotton wool dipped in warm soapy water. Always wipe backwards, pushing any bowel motions away from the birth area. Finally, tell the mother to keep her mouth open and *pant* with her pains, so that she does not push down on the baby.

From now on, let Nature take its course. Don't pull on the baby or the cord. In fact, don't interfere at all unless the cord is round the baby's neck (in which case, unloop it) or if there is a membrane across his face (in which case, tear it away).

The head is normally born first. Support it gently in your hands until the shoulders are born, when you can hook your fingers under the armpits and gently support the chest. Remember that the child will be very slippery and ease him gently into a clean warm towel laid across the mother's thigh.

Once the baby is wrapped in his towel, hold him *carefully* upside down to drain fluid from his mouth and throat. Use a clean piece of cotton wool to wipe blood and mucus from the lips and nose. Lie him on his side, and wait.

The baby should start crying within a minute or so. If he doesn't *don't* smack him. Make sure his mouth is clear, and then *very* gently give the 'kiss of life' as described under FIRST AID TECHNIQUES OF RESUSCITATION. Only blow in as much air as you can hold in your cheeks.

THE CORD. The dangers of interfering with the afterbirth (placenta) and the cord are so great that it's best to leave them entirely alone unless you are a nurse or have proper first aid training.

Simply leave the baby lying on his side by the mother (still, of course, attached to her by the cord) until her pains

return briefly and she pushes the afterbirth out. (Make sure that the blood and fluid that often accompany this do not go into the baby's mouth or nose.)

Place the afterbirth and cord in the cot with the baby. In due course, you may be able to find a nurse who knows how to cut the cord safely, but there is no hurry. Hopefully, by this time the ambulance would have arrived!

Keep the mother warm and lying flat, and encourage her to sleep.

R

RESUSCITATION (*See* FIRST AID TECHNIQUES OF RESUSCITATION.)

S

STINGS

Commonly encountered stings are caused by insects, jellyfish and plants. (Snake 'stings' are dealt with under SNAKE BITE in the A–Z of Conditions.)

Insect Stings

BEE STINGS. These are rarely serious. If the sting is still in the skin, remove it gently with a pair of tweezers or the blade of a knife. Don't squeeze the skin. In fact, if you leave things completely alone, after removing the sting, the inflammation should soon be gone. Occasionally, the pain may be quite severe—if so, apply a pad of cotton wool dipped in cold water to the skin and take some aspirin. Wasp-Eze or PR Spray (see below) may well help in relieving pain.

In cases of multiple bee stings (which may happen if a whole swarm of bees attacks somebody) or stings in the mouth, always see a doctor as soon as possible.

A small number of people are allergic to bee stings, and in such patients collapse and even sudden death may occur after a single sting. If a person who has been stung collapses, rush him to hospital, and be prepared to give the 'kiss of life' (as described under FIRST AID TECHNIQUES OF RESUSCITATION) if breathing stops.

WASP STINGS. These too, are usually fairly trivial. Consult a doctor immediately, however, if the sting is in the mouth as the swelling could block the throat. There is no actual sting to remove from the skin.

Cold compresses and aspirin can be used to relieve pain. It's traditional to put mild acids (vinegar or lemon juice) on wasp stings, and mild alkalis (such as bicarbonate of soda) on bee-stings but there's no evidence at all that this is helpful.

But three fairly new pain-relieving sprays, Wasp-Eze, Burn-Eze and PR Spray may help a bit. You don't need a prescription to get them from a chemist.

If collapse occurs treat as described under bee stings, above. (*See also* INSECT BITES in the A–Z of Conditions.)

Jelly-fish Stings

Wash the skin gently with water to remove any pieces of jelly-fish still adhering. No further treatment is required for trivial injuries, but any extensive sting with a widened area of reddened or blistered skin needs medical treatment. Muscle cramps, weakness and collapse may occur after a sting by the Portuguese Man-o'-War (the jelly-fish which can be identified by the inflated bladder which it puts up as a 'sail'). Any patient stung by this creature should be taken to a doctor as soon as possible.

Nettle Stings

Even the severest nettle stings pass off within a few hours. The traditional treatment with a cool dock leaf is quite satisfactory, though a cold compress will be more effective. A quick burst of Wasp-Eze or PR Spray will be soothing.

Other Stings

The stings of exotic creatures (centipedes, scorpions and so on) are rarely quite as dangerous as people imagine, but may sometimes be serious, especially where children are concerned. Always take the patient straight to a local doctor, who will be familiar with the possible effects of the sting and the correct method of treatment.

U

UNCONSCIOUSNESS
First Aid in Cases of Unconsciousness

The immediate danger is that the patient may choke to death, particularly if his tongue falls back into his throat and blocks his airway. Immediately turn him onto his side, in the 'coma' position or Recovery Position. If you turn him on his right side, bend his left arm and leg upward so that they support him and place the right arm behind his back.

Clear his mouth of anything that may be blocking it (blood clot, vomit, etc.) as quickly as possible. Take out any dentures, and loosen the collar, so that there is no constriction round the neck.

Next, check to make sure there is no bleeding. If there is, control it (*see* BLEEDING). Assuming that the patient is breathing, your next job is to call an ambulance—in fact, it's better if you can get somebody else to do it while you stay with the patient.

If breathing stops, give the 'kiss of life'. If the heart stops, give cardiac massage. Both procedures are described under FIRST AID TECHNIQUES OF RESUSCITATION.

Fainting

Of course, many (perhaps most) cases of unconsciousness are simply due to fainting. This is a particularly likely cause where the patient is young and healthy, or where he or she has been standing for a long time, or has just got up from a chair.

FIRST AID. Don't sit the patient up or try to force brandy or other drinks down the throat. Turn him or her on their side and make sure the airway is clear as described above. In an ordinary faint, recovery will take place within half a minute, provided the patient is allowed to lie flat. The only danger occurs if well-meaning people drag the victim upright.

After regaining consciousness, the person who has fainted should preferably lie down for half an hour. It's best to take things easy for the rest of the day.

W

WASP STINGS (*See* STINGS.)

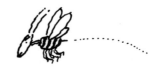

INDEX

Entries which are listed as main headings are followed by numerals in **bold**.

Abdominal pain 31, **42**
Abortion 7, **42–3**
Abrasions **43**
Abscesses 32, **43**
Acne **43–4**, 98
Acupuncture **44**
Adenoids **30**, 113
Adolescence 24
Alcoholism 16, **44–5**
Allergies **45**, 105
Alopecia **45–6**
Amnesia **46**
Amphetamine abuse **46**, 52
Anaemia 14, **46–7**, 66, 95
   pernicious **96**
   in pregnancy 101
   in rheumatoid arthritis 107
   sickle cell **112**
Anal eczema 102
Anal pruritus 102
Angina **47**
Ankle, sprained 114
Ankylosing spondylitis **47**, 48, 50
Antidepressants 26, 64, 84
Anxiety 25, 26, 89
Appendicitis 42, **47**, 119, 130
Arteries **30**
Arteriosclerosis 30
Arthritis (Arthrosis) **47–8**
Ascites 67
Aspirin abuse and poisoning 48
Asthma 45, **48–9**, 68, 72
Atheroma 30
Athlete's foot **49**
Autism **49–50**

Babies **18–19**
   diarrhoea in 19, 65–6
   jaundiced 85, 106
   rashes in 105
   rhesus 105–6
Backache **50**; in pregnancy 101
Bad breath **50–1**
Baldness 45–6, **51**
Barber's itch **51**
Barbiturates, abuse and poisoning **51–2**
Bat ears **52**
BCG (anti-TB) vaccine 23
Bedsores **52**
Bed-wetting **52–3**
Bee stings 140
Bell's palsy **53**
Benign growths 76
Birthmarks **53**
Black 'hairy' tongue 123
Black motions 31
Black vomit 19, 131
Blackheads **53**
Bladder **30**
Bleeding
   emergencies and first aid **133**

from the bowel 31
vaginal 40; in pregnancy 101
Blood pressure **53–4**. *See also*
   High blood pressure
Boils **54**
Bowels **30–1**, 56, 59, 61
Brain **31–2**
Breast **32–4**
Breastfeeding 19
Breath-holding attacks **133–4**
Bronchiectasis **54**
Bronchiolitis **54**
Bronchitis **54–5**, 68, 119
Bronchopneumonia 98
Brucellosis **55**
Bruises **55**
Bunion **55**, 76
Burns, first aid for **134**

Cancer 7, **55–6**
   of the bowel 31, 56
   of the breast 32–3, 56
   cervical 34, 56
   of the gullet 56
   of the larynx 56
   lung 7, 16, 121
   of the prostate 38, 56
   of the skin 56
   of the stomach 56
   of the womb 41, 56
Cannabis (Pot) usage **56**, 78
Carbohydrates in diet 14
Carbuncle **56**
Cardiac massage **136–7**
Cardiomyopathies 78
Cartilage injuries **56–7**, 85
Cataracts **57**
Catarrh **57**
Cavernous haemangiomas 53
'Central' vomiting 131
Cerebral abscess 32
Cerebral embolism 116
Cerbral haemorrhage 116
Cerebral palsy 113
Cerebral thrombosis 116
Cerebral tumour 39, 69
Cervical erosion 34, 41, 89
Cervicitis 34, 41
Cervix **34**
Chest pain **57**
Chicken pox **57**, 104, 105, 111, 119
Child Health Clinic 11
Childhood **20–2**
Choking, first aid for **134**
Cholecystitis 36
Cholera **58**
Chronic bronchitis 54–5, 68, 121
Cirrhosis of the liver 45, **58**
Cleft palate **58**, 76
Clotting thrombosis 97
Coeliac disease **58**, 66
Colds 22, **58–9**, 119
Colic **59**
Community Health Service 11
Colostomy **59**
Colour blindness **59**
Concussion 31
Congenital heart disease 78

Conjunctivitis **59–60**
Constipation **60**
Convulsions 19, 69, 119, **134**
Corns **60**
Coronary heart disease 78, 121
Coronary thrombosis 57, **60–1**, 78, 103, **134**
Cough 22, **61**
Cretinism 40
Crohn's disease **61**
Croup **61**
Cystic fibrosis **61–2**
Cystitis 30, 36, 38, 42, **62**, 103

Da Costa's syndrome 94
Dandruff **62**
Deafness 21, **62–3**, 68, 88, 94
Death Cap fungus 121
Dentist, your family 10
Depression 25, 26, 27, 32, **63–4**, 83, 89, 111
Desensitization 82
Diabetes insipidus **64**
➤ Diabetes mellitus **64–5**, 82, 102, 103
Diarrhoea 22, **65–6**, 72, 73
Diet, a healthy 14
Dieting 71
Diphtheria 7, **66**
Dislocations **66**
Diverticular disease 42, **66**
Dizziness 32, **66**
Doctor, your family **9–10**
Dog bites **135**
Dreams **67**
Drinking *see* Alcoholism
Dropsy **67**
Drowning **135**
Drug addiction 24, 69 *and see under individual drugs*
Duodenal ulcer 31, 103, 121, 127–8
Dust allergy 45, 49

Ear **34–5**, 119; wax in the **131**
Earache 22, **67–8**
ECT treatment 64
Ectopic pregnancy 42, **68**
Eczema 45, 49, **68**, 72
Electric shock 87, **135–6**
Emphysema **68**, 121
Encephalitis 32, 88
Endometriosis **69**
Enlarged prostate 38
Epileptic disorders **69–70**, 134
Erysipelas **70**
Exposure 119

Fainting **141**
Fallopian tubes 115
   inflammation of 42, 109
   pregnancy in 68
Family Planning Clinic 11, 15
Fatness **70–1**; in children 21
Fats in diet 14
Fertility problems **114–15**
Fibroids **71**, 76, 81, 89
Fibrositis **71**, 106
Fits 69–70, 134
Flat foot **72**

Flea bites **72**
Food allergies 72
Food poisoning **72–3**
Fractures, first aid for **137**
Fungus poisoning 72
Furred tongue 123

Gall bladder **35–6**, 42
Gall stone 35, 116
   colic 35, 59
   jaundice 35, 85
Gardnerella vaginalis 41
Gas poisoning **137–8**
Gastrectomy 128
Gastric ulcer 31, 127–8
Gastritis **73**, 130
Gastro-enteritis 42, **73**, 119, 130
Geographical tongue 123
German measles 63, **73–4**, 104, 105, 119
Glandular fever **74**, 119
Glaucoma **74**
Goitre 39, **74**
Gonorrhoea **74–5**, 93, 118
Gout **75**
Grand mal 69
Grave's disease 39
Groin hernia 107–8
Growing pains **75**
Growths **76**
Gum disorders **76**

Haemoptysis 61, 114
Haemorrhoids *see* Piles
Halitosis *see* Bad breath
Hallucinations 28, **76**
Hallux valgus **76**
Hammer toe **76**
Hangnails 92
Hard sores 122
Hare lip 58, **76**
Hay fever 45, 49, 57, **76–7**
Head injuries 31; first aid for **138**
Headache **77**
Heart attacks 7, 30, 60–1, **134**
Heart failure **77**
Heart trouble 27, **77–8**
Heartburn **78**
Heimlich's manoeuvre 134
Hepatitis (infective and serum) 84–5
Hernia **107–9**
Heroin addiction 78–9, 90
Herpes 41, 130
Hiatus hernia **79**
Hiccup **79**
High blood pressure 53–4, 94, 103, 116
'Hives' 72, 128
Hodgkin's disease **79**
Homosexuality **79–80**
Hospital service **10–11**
Hot flushes 27, 81, 89
Housemaid's knee **80**
Huntington's disease 109
Hydrocephalus **80**
Hyperemesis 102
Hypertension *see* High blood pressure

Hyperthyroidism 39
Hypothermia 7, **80–1**, 119
Hysterectomy 41, 71, **81**, 90
Hysteria 25, **81** 132

Immunizations 19, 20, 23, 128
Impetigo **81**
Impotence **81–2**
Incisional hernia 108–9
Indigestion **82**
Influenza **82–3**, 119
Ingrowing toenail **122**
Insect bites, stings **83**, 140–1
Insomnia **83–4**
Intercourse, difficulties in **84**
Iron deficiency anaemia 14, 46–7
Itching **84**, 102

Jaundice **84–5**
Jelly-fish stings 141

Keeping fit in middle age 27
'Keloid' **110**
Kidney stones 37, 59, 116
Kidneys **36–7**, 53, 62, 103
'Kiss of life' **136**
Knee injuries 56–7, **85**, 114
Knock knee **85**

Labour, stages of **138**
Laryngitis **85–6**, 119
Lead poisoning **86**
Legionnaires' disease **86**
Lesbianism **86**
Leukaemia **86–7**
Lice infestation **87**
Ligaments, torn 85
Lightning, injuries from **87**
Liver 37
Lobar pneumonia 99
Lockjaw (tetanus) 43, **87**
Loving, importance of 15
Lumbago **87**, 106
Lumps **87**
Lung cancer 7, 16, 121
Lung TB 124–5
Lungs 37

Malignant growths 76. *See also*
  Cancer
Mandrax abuse **88**
Mastitis 33
Masturbation **88**
Measles 7, 20, **88**, 105, 119
Meniere's disease **88–9**, 131
Meningitis 32, 77, **89**
Menopause 26–7, 81, **89**
Mental illness **89–90**
Metropathia **90**
Middle age 26–7
Migraine 77, **90**, 131
Miscarriage **90**, 101
Moles 53, 56
'Monkeypox' 112
Morning sickness 102, 130
Morphine addiction **90**
Mouth ulcers 76, 122–3, 127
Multiple sclerosis **91**

Mumps **91–2**, 104, 119
Myxoedema 40

Nail disorders **92**
Nappy rash **92–3**
Nausea **93**
National Health Service **9**
Nephritis 36
'Nerves', nervousness **93**
'Nettle rash' 128
Nettle stings 141
Neuralgia **93**, 111
Neurosis **93**
Nightmares 67
Non-specific urethritis (NSU)
  93–4, 118
Nosebleeds **94**

Obesity *see* Fatness
Oedema 67
Old age 27–8
Opium addiction **94**
Orchitis 91
Osteoarthritis 48, 50, 57, 85, 106
Otosclerosis 63, **94**
Ovulation 96

Palpitations **94**
Papillomas 76
Papular urticaria 83
Paratyphoid 126
Parkinson's disease **95**
Paronychia 92
Peptic ulcers 127–8
Perennial rhinitis 76
Periods, period problems 89, **95–6**
Pernicious anaemia **96**
Pertussis 131
Perversion **96–7**
Petit mal 69
Pharyngitis 113
Phenacetin abuse **97**
Phenylketonuria **97**
Phlebitis **97**, 120
Piles 31, **97–8**, 102, 105, 128
Pimples **98**
Pituitary gland 64
Placenta praevia **98**, 101
Pleurisy 57, **98**
Pneumoconiosis 68, **98**, 112
Pneumonia 88, **98–9**, 119
Pneumothorax **99**
Poisoning, first aid for **139**
Polio 7, 19, 20, **99**
Pollen allergy 49, 76
Polyps of the cervix 34, 41
'Port wine stains' 53
Pot smoking *see* Cannabis
Pre-eclampsia 101, 139
Pregnancy 18, **99–102**
  ectopic 42, **68**
  twin **125–6**
  unwanted 24
Prematurity 100, 126, **139–40**
Prolapse of the womb 41
Prostate gland **37–8**
Protein in diet 14
Pruritus **102**

Psoriasis **102**
Psychosomatic disorders 94, **102–3**
Puberty 23–4
Pulmonary embolism 57, **103**, 120
Pulmonary tuberculosis 124–5
Pyelitis 36, 42, **103**, 119
Pyelonephritis 36, **103**
Pyloric stenosis **103**

Quarantine **104**
Quinsy **104**

Rabies **104**, 135
Rashes **104–5**
Rectal disorders **105**
Relaxation, importance of 15
Renal colic 42
Retention of urine 38, **105**, 116
Retirement, coping with 28
Rhesus factor **105–6**
Rheumatic fever **106**
Rheumatic heart disease 78
Rheumatism 26, **106**
Rheumatoid arthritis 48, **106–7**, 115
Rickets **107**
Ringworm 45, 102, **107**
Rodent ulcer **107**, 127
Rubella vaccine 23
'Run-around' 92, 122
Rupture (hernia) **107–9**

St Vitus' dance **109**
Salmonella germs 72, 126
Salpingitis 42, **109**
Scabies 84, **109**
Scalds **110**
Scarlet fever (Scarlatina) **110**
Scars **110**
Schizophrenia **110**
Schoolchildren 22–4
  rashes in 105
Sciatica 106, **110–11**
Scurvy 76, **111**
Sea-sickness 124
Sebaceous cyst **111**
Senile dementia 27, 32
Sex 15
Sexual infections 15–16. *See also*
  Venereal diseases
Shingles 93, 104, **111**
Shock **111–12**, 134
Sickle cell anaemia **112**
Silicosis **112**
Sinusitis 77, **112**
Skin cancer 56
Skin ulcers 56, 127
Sleep 15
Sleeping pills 28, 51, 88
'Slipped disc' 50
Smallpox 104, 105, **112–13**
Smoking 7, 16. *See also* Tobacco
  addiction
Snake bite **113**
Snoring **113**
Sore throat **113**, 119
Spastic disorders **113–14**
Spleen **38–9**
Sprains **114**

Sputum **114**
Squint **114**
Stammering **114**
Staphylococci poisoning 72
Sterility **114–15**
Sterilization **115**
Still's disease **115–16**
Stings **140–1**
Stomach cancer 56
Stones **116**. *See* Gall stones,
  Kidney stones
'Storkmarks' 53
'Strawberry marks' 53
Stress 15, 26, 103
Stricture **116**
Strokes 30, 32, 54, 69, 103, **116**, 134
Styes **116–17**
Sub-arachnoid haemorrhage **117**
Suicide 64
Sunburn **117–18**
Sunstroke **117–18**
Sydenham's chorea 109
Syphilis **118**

Temperature, raised or low **118–20**
'Test tube babies' 115
Tetanus *see* Lockjaw
Threadworms 102
Thrombosis **120**
Thrush 41, 102, **120**
Thyroid gland **39–40**
Thyrotoxicosis 39
Tic douloureux 93, 120
Tics **120–1**
Toadstool poisoning **121**
Tobacco addiction 16, **121–2**
Toenail, ingrowing **122**
Tongue disorders **122–3**
Tonsils, tonsillitis 22, 110, 119, **123**,
  130
Toothache **123**
Toxaemia 101, 126, 139
Travel sickness **124**, 131
Trichomonas vaginalis 41, 102, **124**
Tuberculosis 37, 109, **124–5**
Tummy upsets 22. *See* Diarrhoea
  etc.
Tumours **125**
  brain 32
  cerebral 39, 69
Twin pregnancy **125–6**
Typhoid fever **126–7**

Ulcerative colitis 65, 128
Ulcers 42, **127–8**, 130, 131
  varicose 129
Umbilical hernia 108
Unconsciousness **141**
Undulant fever 55
Urticaria 72, **128**
  papular 83

Vaccination **128**
Vagina **40–1**
  irritation and discharge 40–1,
  102, 120
Vagotomy 128
Varicose veins 120, **128–9**

Vascular brain disorders 31–2
Vasectomy **129**
Vein thrombosis 120
Venereal diseases 11, 15–16, 24, 74–5, 93–4, 109, 118, **129–30**
Verruca **130**
Vertigo 66, 88, **130**, 131

Vitamin deficiency 130
Vomiting 22, **130–1**
  in babies 19
  in pregnancy 102
Vulval irritation 102

Warts 130, **131**

Wasp sting 141
'Water on the brain' 80
Wax in the ears **131**
'Wen' 111
'Wet dreams' 67
Whitlow 92, 122
Whooping cough 19, 104, 119, **131–2**

Wind **132**
Womb **41**
Worms **132**
Wrist injuries 114, **132**
Wry neck **132**

ACKNOWLEDGEMENTS

Designer: Harry Green
Artists: Paula Youens
        Oxford Illustrators

The author and the publishers are grateful to the following for permission to reproduce their photographs:
pages *2, 6, 11, 12, 14, 20, 23, 25, 26, 27, 121* Richard & Sally Greenhill; *8* and *100* Pictorial Press; *17, 18* and *22* Graham Portlock; *33* Black Star; *39, 71, 133* and *137* Camera Press; *104* Keystone Press.